TABLE OF CONTENTS

EXECUTIVE SUMMARY

Background

Fragile X syndrome (FXS), caused by a mutation in a specific gene on the X chromosome, is the most common inherited cause of intellectual and developmental disabilities (IDD). Variation within the same gene has been linked to Fragile X-associated Tremor/Ataxia Syndrome (FXTAS), a tremor/ataxia disorder occurring primarily in older men, and Fragile X-associated Primary Ovarian Insufficiency (FXPOI), generally identified in woman of child bearing age. Collectively, FXS, FXTAS, and FXPOI represent a major health burden and have far-reaching implications for individuals, families, and their future generations.

Charge to Working Groups

In the spring of 2008 the National Institutes of Health (NIH) convened working groups charged with developing comprehensive recommendations for specific, high-priority research objectives for FXS and the associated disorders of FXTAS and FXPOI. The working groups were composed of scientific experts from the research and clinical communities, along with representatives for affected individuals and family members, other pertinent federal agencies and invested NIH Institutes and Centers (ICs). The goals were designed to be used by the NIH and FXS, FXTAS, and FXPOI research communities and to be shared with other federal agencies to facilitate coordinated research activities that will lead to timely detection, diagnosis, treatment, and prevention of the targeted disorders.

Research Goals

The research goals that follow were generated by the disorder-specific working groups. Specific objectives for each of the goals are discussed in detail within the *Research Plan on Fragile X Syndrome and Associated Disorders*. The goals are grouped by disorder and are not listed by order of importance.

Fragile X Syndrome (FXS)
Goal I. Advance the understanding of the pathophysiology of FXS.
Goal II. Improve appropriate and timely diagnosis of individuals with FXS by conducting population-based screens.
Goal III. Validate and use functional measures of the manifestation of FXS across the life span.
Goal IV. Initiate a broad-based program of research on the efficacy of treatments of FXS.
Goal V. Advance the understanding of the ramifications of FXS for families.
Goal VI. Create an FXS research infrastructure and resources to maximize research efficiencies and promote large-scale research collaborations.

Fragile X-associated Tremor/Ataxia Syndrome (FXTAS)
Goal I. Define pathogenic mechanisms of FXTAS.
Goal II. Define clinical phenotypes of FXTAS.

Goal II. Gain a better understanding of the epidemiology of FXTAS and premutation alleles.
Goal IV. Develop means of early diagnosis/identification of individuals most at risk of developing FXTAS.
Goal V. Develop supportive and targeted therapeutic interventions for FXTAS.
Goal VI. Examine quality-of-life issues associated with FXTAS.
Goal VII. Explore broader implications for other neurodegenerative diseases.
Goal VIII. Establish a general research infrastructure for FXTAS.

Fragile X-associated Primary Ovarian Insufficiency (FXPOI)
Goal I. Examine FXPOI disease-specific mechanisms and therapeutic targets.
Goal II. Examine FXPOI disease progression and preventive medicine.
Goal III. Examine genetic and environmental factors that influence the onset and severity of FXPOI.
Goal IV. Examine the diagnosis, treatment, and management of FXPOI.
Goal V. Establish FXPOI specific infrastructure needs.

INTRODUCTION

In its report in the fiscal year 2008 budget for the U.S. Department of Health and Human Services (DHHS), the Senate Committee on Appropriations requested that *the NIH, through the NICHD* [the *Eunice Kennedy Shriver* National Institute of Child Health and Human Development] *and other participating Institutes, convene a scientific session in 2008 to develop pathways to new opportunities for collaborative, directed research across Institutes, and to produce a blueprint of coordinated research strategies and public-private partnership opportunities for Fragile X.*" The NIH Fragile X Research Coordinating Group (formed in March 2007) assumed the task of bringing together representatives from the research and clinical communities along with representatives for affected individuals and family members and other pertinent federal agencies. Three working groups, one for each of the primary disorders associated with Fragile X syndrome (FXS), were formed in March of 2008 and charged with developing comprehensive recommendations for specific high-priority research objectives for FXS and the associated disorders of Fragile X-associated Tremor/Ataxia Syndrome (FXTAS) and Fragile X-associated Primary Ovarian Insufficiency (FXPOI). The goals were designed to be used by the NIH and the FXS, FXTAS, and FXPOI research communities and to be shared with other federal agencies to facilitate coordinated research activities that will lead to timely detection, diagnosis, treatment, and prevention of the targeted disorders.

FXS and Associated Disorders — Overview

FMR1 and FMRP

> **Gene Terminology**
> *FMR1* – refers to the human gene
> *Fmr1* – refers to the mouse gene
> *dfmr1* – refers to the fly gene

The "Fragile X Mental Retardation 1" gene (*FMR1*) was named for its location on the X chromosome and its characteristic fragile appearance under the microscope under certain conditions when mutated. Three primary disorders have been associated with mutations of the *FMR1* gene: FXS, FXTAS, and FXPOI. Although the three disorders have very different clinical symptoms, they all result from variations in a region of the *FMR1* gene that contains multiple repeats of three nucleotides, the individual building blocks of DNA. A number of other diseases are also caused by such trinucleotide repeats in other genes. In the case of *FMR1*-associated disorders, the specific repeated pattern is cytosine-guanine-guanine (CGG), and differences in the number of CGG repeats in the gene determine the three most common forms of the gene: normal, premutation, and full mutation.

Individuals with fewer than ~55 repeats have a normal *FMR1* gene. Individuals with more than 200 repeats have a full mutation and FXS. The full mutation leads to a silencing of the gene through methylation and chromatin changes that lead to a deficiency of the Fragile X Mental Retardation Protein (FMRP). FMRP functions as an RNA-binding protein that appears to regulate the production of proteins from specific messenger RNAs, which are important for the creation and proper maintenance of synaptic connections between neurons in the central nervous system. Full mutations are generally associated with intellectual and development disabilities (IDD) apparent in early childhood. Repeats in the range of ~55 to 200 are called "premutations" and are associated with two primary adult-onset disorders: FXTAS and FXPOI. In addition to carrying a risk for later developing FXTAS and FXPOI, premutation carriers may show clinical symptoms as children. These include attention-deficit hyperactivity disorder (ADHD), anxiety, shyness, social deficits, and, on occasion, autism-spectrum disorders; boys appear to be more often affected than girls.

FMR1-associated disorders are heritable, and carriers of the premutation can transmit expanded forms of the gene to their children. As an unstable gene, there is also the risk that a premutation may expand to full mutation during transmission. The risk for the expansion of repeats during transmission depends on the premutation size and the parental origin. Among female carriers, a repeat length of ~100 or greater has almost a 100-percent chance of expanding to a full mutation in one generation, while repeat lengths of 70 to 79 have about a 30 percent chance. For repeat lengths of 45 to 54, expansion to a full mutation is unlikely in one generation, but the risk increases after several generations. When passed down through the father, the premutation repeat length is more stable and rarely, if at all, expands to a full mutation.

Collectively, the *FMR1*-associated disorders of FXS, FXTAS, and FXPOI represent a major health burden and have far-reaching implications for individuals, families, and their future generations. Each of the disorders is described more fully in the following sections.

Fragile X Syndrome (FXS)

FXS is the most common inherited cause of IDD and has been estimated to occur in approximately 1 in 2,500 males and females across all racial and ethnic groups. IDD in FXS ranges from mild to severe, and females are more mildly affected, on average, than males because of X inactivation on the single X chromosome in males. Emotional and behavioral problems, including attention problems, hyperactivity, anxiety, mood instability, tantrums, aggression, and social deficits, are common. As many as 30 to 50 percent of individuals with FXS meet the diagnostic criteria for autism or autism spectrum disorders (ASDs). FXS is considered a portal for understanding a variety of neurobehavioral disorders, including autism, ADHD, and anxiety disorders.

In FXS, the lack of FMRP leads to alterations in protein synthesis throughout the brain, as FMRP appears to be involved in a number of translational activities. Recent research shows that a number of key pathways are dysregulated in the absence of FMRP. These findings have led to the experimental use of medications to reverse the signaling and synaptic abnormalities seen in animal models of FXS, and human clinical trials have been initiated to test the possibility of reversing or decreasing the severity of IDD and behavioral problems. Research on several biomarkers is currently ongoing and could provide important information for treating FXS and other developmental disorders.

Fragile X-associated Tremor/Ataxia Syndrome (FXTAS)

FXTAS is the most severe form of clinical involvement associated with premutation *FMR1* alleles. Its core features are intention tremor and/or ataxia, with lower-extremity neuropathy, autonomic dysfunction, and gradual cognitive decline beginning with memory and executive function deficits. Psychiatric features including anxiety, dysinhibition, depression, and apathy are also common problems. Associated clinical features include peripheral neuropathy, dysautonomia, and particularly in women with FXTAS, hypothyroidism and muscle pain/fibromyalgia. Symptoms of FXTAS typically appear after age 50, although the age of onset correlates with the CGG expansion within the premutation range — the higher the number of repeats, the earlier the onset of tremor or ataxia. The penetrance of FXTAS is incomplete, meaning that not all carriers develop symptoms, and men are more commonly affected than women. Preliminary data on life expectancy from age of onset are variable, with a range from five to 25 years.

Both males and females with FXTAS display the characteristic neuropathological feature of exclusively intranuclear spherical particles (inclusions) in neurons and astrocytes. The density of the inclusions throughout the central nervous system (CNS) correlates with the size of the CGG repeat expansion. Brain imaging of FXTAS with magnetic resonance imaging (MRI) globally shows brain atrophy, white matter disease in subcortical, middle cerebellar peduncles (MCP) and periventricular regions, and dilated ventricles.

Numerous lines of evidence from cell-, animal-, and human-based investigations point to an RNA "toxic" gain of function as the pathogenic basis of FXTAS: First, the disorder is largely confined to carriers of active premutation alleles of the *FMR1* gene. Second, *FMR1* gene expression is abnormal in that *FMR1* mRNA levels are elevated by as much as eightfold; the mRNA itself is altered due to the presence of the expanded CGG repeat. Third, both mouse and fruit fly *(Drosophila)* models that harbor premutation CGG-repeat expansions (~90 to 100 CGG repeats), even without the coding portion of the *FMR1* gene, manifest features of the neuropathology of FXTAS.

It should be emphasized that the neurodegenerative disorder, FXTAS, and the neurodevelopmental disorder, FXS, are completely different clinical syndromes in whom they affect (premutation carriers vs. carriers of full-mutation alleles), age ranges of onset (late adult vs. childhood), and mechanism of pathogenesis (RNA toxicity due to increased gene expression vs. absence of protein due to gene silencing). This distinction is often unrecognized among members of the health profession.

The development of therapeutic approaches for many late-onset neurodegenerative disorders (e.g., late-onset Parkinson and Alzheimer disease) has been complicated by their generally sporadic nature, which largely precludes the identification of clear pathogenesis-phenotype relationships. As a late-onset neurodegenerative disorder with a known pathogenic trigger, FXTAS represents an important tool for understanding global mechanisms of neurodegeneration.

Fragile X-associated Primary Ovarian Insufficiency (FXPOI)

Women with the fragile X premutation are at risk for premature ovarian failure (POF) or primary ovarian insufficiency (POI), which is the onset of menopausal symptoms before the age of 40 years. The term "premature ovarian failure" is often used, but the disorder can be better described as "primary ovarian insufficiency." POI reflects the continuum of ovarian dysfunction that ends with POF. However, POI encompasses the entire spectrum leading up to POF, which has been determined to include the first sign of infertility, regular menstrual cycles with an elevated follicle-stimulating hormone (FSH) level (indicating decreased ovarian follicles), and irregular menstrual cycles through the final menstrual period. Regardless of cause, women with POI not only experience loss of normal fertility but are also at increased risk for osteoporosis and cardiac disease and have higher rates of mortality. Thus, women who have a fragile X premutation face the increased health risks related to POI and FXTAS as well as the risk that their children will inherit the unstable repeat as either the pre- or full mutation.

This report refers to the ovarian dysfunction as "Fragile X-associated Primary Ovarian Insufficiency (FXPOI)," to reflect the continuum of ovarian function and the association with fragile X-associated disorders. Fragile X premutation carriers, as a group, experience menopause approximately five years earlier than normal women, and analysis of hormones in women with the premutation who still have regular menstrual cycles shows indications of early ovarian aging. While the rate of POI is low in the general population (1 percent), women with the premutation ascertained through families with FXS have up to a 24-percent rate of POI. The carrier frequency of the fragile X premutation in women in the general population is estimated to be around 1/130. However, in women who are experiencing POI, the prevalence ranges from 1/33 in isolated cases to 1/8 in women who have a positive family history of POI. Therefore, detecting this common triplet repeat disorder is one of the most fruitful means of identifying women at risk for POI and represents an important opportunity to increase knowledge regarding the underlying biological mechanism leading to POI. Additionally, because 20 percent of couples presenting to infertility practices show evidence of POI, it would be important to screen for the fragile X premutation in infertility patients to help develop tailored treatment strategies.

Despite its clinical importance, POI cannot be predicted in a majority of cases, nor can the longitudinal course of ovarian function be defined. Most often, a woman diagnosed with POI has few treatment options. Women who carry the fragile X premutation therefore provide an important window to further study mechanisms of POI. Genetic testing for fragile X premutations offers a unique opportunity to identify women at risk for POI and to study the risk factors and longitudinal course of the disease. Increased knowledge regarding the course of FXPOI may lead to improved health care for women experiencing POI from *FMR1* mutations as well as other causes.

There is no recommended standard of care for a woman carrying the fragile X premutation with respect to her prognosis for a shortened reproductive life span. Determining the risk factors and time course of the reproductive abnormalities associated with the fragile X premutation could have an enormous impact on counseling about prognosis, fertility potential, fertility treatment, and risks for FXS and could help define recommendations for testing and fertility preservation. From a broader health perspective, the time course could also impact counseling regarding the risks of osteoporosis and cardiovascular disease.

NIH FRAGILE X AND ASSOCIATED DISORDERS RESEARCH ACTIVITIES

The NIH Fragile X Research Coordinating Group (FXRCG)

Over the past several years, research programs with support from across NIH have made significant advances in the understanding of FXS and the associated disorders of FXTAS and FXPOI. While a number of NIH ICs have supported research relating to these disorders, the coordination of research efforts was informal until recently. In January 2007, the Director of the NICHD established the FXRCG to encourage coordinated research efforts and facilitate collaboration across NIH and with other federal agencies and advocacy groups. Participants were nominated by Institute directors at the invitation of the NICHD.

The coordinating group is composed of NIH extramural staff and intramural researchers at Institutes that support and conduct research projects related to FXS and the associated disorders of FXTAS and FXPOI. These Institutes include: the NICHD, the National Institute of Mental Health (NIMH), the National Institute of Neurological Disorders and Stroke (NINDS) the National Institute on Aging (NIA), the National Institute of Diabetes and Digestive and Kidney Diseases (NIDDK), the National Institute of General Medical Sciences [NIGMS], the National Cancer Institute (NCI), and the National Institute on Deafness and Other Communication Disorders (NIDCD). In March 2007 the coordinating group met for the first time and shared a review of research activities currently conducted and supported by the NIH.

NIH Fragile X Research Coordinating Group Membership

Tiina K. Urv, Ph.D., Health Scientist Administrator, NICHD (GROUP CHAIR)

Cara Allen, Ph.D., Health Science Policy Analyst, NINDS

Richard Anderson, M.D., Ph.D., Program Director, NIGMS

Andrea Beckel-Mitchener, Ph.D., Chief, Functional Neurogenomics Program, NIMH

Dana Bynum, Psychologist, Referral & Program Analysis Branch, NICHD

Diane Cooper, Informationist, Division of Library Services, NIH Library

George Gaines, Chief, Office of Program and Public Liaison, NICHD

Lisa Gilotty, Ph.D., Chief, Social Behavior and Autism Program, NIMH

Lawrence Nelson, M.D., Division of Intramural Research, NICHD

Michele Pearson, Program Analyst, NIMH

Robert Riddle, Ph.D., Program Director, Neurogenetics Cluster, NINDS

David Schlessinger, Ph.D., Laboratory Chief, NIA

Christina Stile, Writer-Editor, NICHD

Stephen Snyder, Program Director, NIA

Margaret Tucker, MD, Director Human Genetics Program, NCI

Susan Taymans, Ph.D., Program Director NICHD

Karen Usdin, Ph.D., Senior Investigator, NIDDK

Bracie Watson, Program Director, Hearing Division of Scientific Programs, NIDCD

Highlights of Ongoing Research at the NIH on FXS and Associated Disorders

A number of NIH ICs have a longstanding history of supporting research relating to FXS and the associated disorders of FXTAS and FXPOI. Current research activities of the ICs with significant portfolios in these areas are summarized below beginning with collaborative efforts that cross ICs and include public-private partnerships.

NIH Collaborative Efforts

The NIH has continuously supported annual conferences on FXS held at Cold Spring Harbor Laboratory's Banbury Conference Center since 2001. With primary support from the NIMH and joint funding from the NICHD and FRAXA—the Fragile X Research Foundation (FRAXA), this highly successful conference focuses on basic and clinical research relevant to FXS. The conference brings together a broad range of scientists, both those working on FXS and others in allied or relevant fields, to share recent research findings and explore additional collaborations.

Through the NIH Common Fund, the NIA, the National center for Research Resources (NCRR), and the NINDS support the Neurotherapeutics Research Consortium, which began in 2007 as an interdisciplinary approach aimed at developing targeted molecular therapeutics for neurogenetic disorders, using FXTAS as its principal research paradigm. The projects supported under the consortium include molecular/cellular neuroscience, animal models, quantitative phenotyping and clinical research, and cognitive neuroscience, all with the common objectives of developing therapeutic interventions and quantitative measures for assessing their efficacy.

There are currently multiple research efforts aimed at developing treatments and novel interventions. One such effort is related to clinical trials of pharmaceuticals for FXS includes an ongoing cooperative agreement led by the NIMH in partnership with the NICHD, NINDS, FRAXA, and Autism Speaks to develop therapeutics related to metabotropic glutamate receptor (mGluR) antagonists to treat FXS and autism. Because of the genetic mutation that causes FXS, individuals with the disorder do not make the protein FMRP. Scientists theorize that, without FMRP, brain cells produce too much of certain other proteins, including those whose production is stimulated by mGluR5, a receptor for the neurotransmitter glutamate. Research in animals suggests that excess production of these other proteins contributes to the weakened connections between brain cells seen in people with FXS. The compounds being developed through the NIH-supported cooperative agreement partially block mGluR5 and were shown to reverse many symptoms associated with the loss of FMRP in mouse models of FXS. This project has been making steady progress, and if further testing confirms the compounds' safety in animals, the scientists will request a U.S. Food and Drug Administration (FDA) permit for research to determine dosage and safety in nonaffected human volunteers before moving forward with clinical trials in people with FXS.

In May of 2008, the NICHD, in collaboration with the Office of Rare Diseases (ORD), NINDS, NIMH, FRAXA, the National Fragile X Foundation (NFXF), and representatives of the Fragile X Clinics Consortium (FXCC), held a two-day scientific meeting to discuss clinical trials with children with FXS. The goal of the meeting was to establish a working group that will develop suggestions related to cognitive and behavioral outcome measures for clinical trials with children with FXS. Participants included members of constituency groups, representatives from the FDA, clinicians who treat children with FXS and researchers with experience in clinical trials of pharmaceuticals with children with FXS. Additional participants included researchers with experience in designing successful clinical trials, psychometric assessments, and in conducting behavioral and cognitive studies of children with FXS. The working group established at this meeting will continue to meet via teleconference to develop suggestions for the field.

The NIH's focus on efforts to understand the relationships between FXS and autism continues through the Program Announcement (PA) soliciting research to study the *Shared Neurobiology of FXS and Autism*. This PA, originally issued in 2005, was reissued in 2007 and remains active. It is a public-private partnership led by the NIMH in collaboration with NINDS and the NICHD. The partnership also includes the Canadian Institutes of Health (Institute of Neurosciences, Mental Health and Addiction and the Institute of Genetics), the Health Research Board of Ireland, FRAXA, the National Alliance for Autism Research, and Autism Speaks. Eleven grants have been awarded through this mechanism since its inception. These studies include a wide array of research ranging from studies examining language in children with FXS to studies in mouse models to explore structural abnormalities in neurons observed in FXS.

National Institute on Aging (NIA)

Most of the FXS-related research supported by the NIA has focused on the disorder FXTAS, an adult-onset (beyond age 50) neurological disorder characterized by gait ataxia and intention tremor that predominately affects older male carriers of the premutation allele in the 5' untranslated region of the *FMR1* gene. Changes in cognition in FXTAS range from mild frontal executive and memory deficits to global dementia. NIA-funded investigations involve mechanistic studies related to inclusion formation, cell loss, brain plasticity and structure, and quantitative measures of CNS dysfunction in FXTAS. The portfolio of grants supported by the NIA examines mainly the cellular and molecular physiology of the synapse and the number and shape of spines that decorate the dendrites forming those synapses. While research on FXS and on FXTAS is important in its own right, the NIA views such efforts as 'instructive' in that the study of these diseases may provide insights into a number of other neurodegenerative diseases associated with the aging brain, including Alzheimer disease.

Eunice Kennedy Shriver National Institute of Child Health and Human Development (NICHD)

The NICHD has funded three Fragile X Research Centers since fiscal year 2003. The Centers, which were originally authorized in the Children's Health Act of 2000, are intended to stimulate the formation of multidisciplinary, multi-institutional teams with a goal of facilitating the translation of basic research findings from "bench-to-bedside-to-community." Research findings from the Centers have helped propel the field of research in FXS and associated disorders forward at a rapid pace. To maintain this momentum of discovery and further develop research relevant to FXS and associated disorders, the NICHD held a successful recompetition in early fiscal year 2008 to fund three Fragile X Research Centers. The three centers include research programs in both basic and clinical science and will be funded late in fiscal year 2008. Several projects will focus on newborn screening, including studies that assess methods of testing immediate and extended family members and the impact of newborn screening on the family.

The NICHD maintains a diverse portfolio of investigator-initiated research related to FXS, FXTAS, and FXPOI that is conducted by both seasoned and new investigators. Clinical studies include examination of the effects of autism on the development of language in children with FXS and the role of visual processing and eye gaze in social and cognitive development. The NICHD also funds numerous projects examining mechanisms and their function involved in FXS.

An area of special interest for the NICHD is newborn screening. The Institute is supporting the development of a screening tool for expanded *FMR1* alleles. The method is applicable for screening both males and females and for allele sizes throughout the premutation (55 to 200 CGG repeats) and full-mutation ranges. The method is capable of rapid detection of expanded alleles using as little as 1 percent of the DNA from a single dried blood spot. The methodology is suitable for screening large populations of newborns or those at high risk (e.g., persons with autism, POI, or ataxia) for expanded *FMR1* alleles.

The NICHD issued a PA entitled *Fragile X Premutation and Ovarian Function* in 2007. This PA encourages investigator-initiated research on basic, clinical, or translational research on the effects of the fragile X premutation on ovarian function, with a focus on POF or early menopause, in women and/or animal models. To date, three applications have been submitted for peer review through this mechanism. This program runs through 2010. The NICHD also funds intramural research related to FXPOI through its Intramural Integrative Reproductive Medicine Unit. This unit is focusing research efforts on spontaneous POI. The unit is also investigating mouse models of POI related to autoimmune oophoritis and the *FMR1* premutation.

National Institute of Diabetes and Digestive and Kidney Diseases (NIDDK)

The intramural program of the NIDDK supports the research of the Gene Structure and Disease section, which studies the *FMR1*-associated disorders. This group is working to understand how the *FMR1* gene becomes silenced in FXS and what can be done to reverse this process. The intramural researchers have recently identified a specific epigenetic change on fragile X alleles that is an important late step in the silencing process. The researchers have also shown that this step can be inhibited quite effectively, thereby allowing the *FMR1* gene to be reactivated in patient cells. They have also developed a mouse model for the *FMR1* associated disorders. Studies using this model system, performed in collaboration with other intramural and extramural clinicians/scientists, will help clarify the biological basis of FXTAS and FXPOI. Working with this model, the research group has also identified two different mutation-associated mechanisms that contribute to the instability of the *FMR1* gene. They have shown that the large maternal mutations that give rise to FXS probably arise from aberrant repair of DNA damage during genesis of egg cells. Identifying the source of the DNA damage may help determine whether there is any possibility of reducing the incidence of the subsequent mutation.

National Institute of Mental Health (NIMH)

In addition to the collaborative PA *Shared Neurobiology of FXS and Autism*, the NIMH has issued a PA entitled *Research on Psychopathology in Intellectual Disabilities*, through which it encourages research designed to elucidate the epidemiology, etiology, treatment, and prevention of mental disorders in persons with IDD, including FXS.

NIMH-funded research on FXS also includes preclinical investigations and studies in patient populations to better understand the processes and biological mechanisms disrupted in FXS. For example, a longitudinal study is examining 120 school-age children with FXS and their families to assess the biological and environmental factors contributing to clinical outcomes. The NIMH continues its support of another longitudinal study, in which researchers are using brain imaging to examine the relationships between the *FMR1* expression, brain abnormalities, and behavior throughout development in a cohort of individuals. Scientists in the NIMH Intramural Research Program are investigating *Fmr1* expression in mouse models of FXS. Early results suggest that there are defects in brain protein synthesis that may underlie disease symptoms. In addition, the NIMH is continuing to support programs focused on training postdoctoral and clinician researchers with an interest in developmental disabilities, including FXS.

National Institute of Neurological Disorders and Stroke (NINDS)

The NINDS supports research to understand how alterations in the *FMR1* gene disrupt neurological development and function, as in FXS and FXTAS, and to ultimately develop treatments or preventive strategies. Research projects related to FXS currently supported by the NINDS include studies on how the FMRP regulates the expression of other proteins in neurons and on its role in a cell-signaling pathway important for learning and memory and known to be disrupted in a mouse model of FXS. The NINDS also supports a training program for research on developmental brain disorders that is associated with one of the NICHD's Fragile X Research Centers.

Research on FXTAS with current support from the NINDS includes a study of how premutation expansions in the *dFmr1* gene lead to neurodegeneration in a fly model of the disorder. It also includes a study of the clinical features and progression of FXTAS using brain imaging and neurological, psychological, and molecular testing in affected individuals, asymptomatic carriers, and healthy subjects without *FMR1* mutations. Along with the NIA and the NCRR, the NINDS also supports the Neurotherapeutics Research Institute, an interdisciplinary consortium funded through the NIH Common Fund that focuses on developing treatments for FXTAS. The two NINDS components are a project to develop mouse models for FXTAS and a clinical study to assess cognitive function in individuals with different sizes of repeat expansions in the *FMR1* gene.

RESEARCH PLAN ON FRAGILE X SYNDROME AND ASSOCIATED DISORDERS

In its report on the fiscal year 2008 budget for the DHHS, the Senate Committee on Appropriations stated:

"The Committee urges the NIH, through the NICHD and other participating Institutes, to convene a scientific session in 2008 to develop pathways to new opportunities for collaborative, directed research across Institutes and to produce a blueprint of coordinated research strategies and public-private partnership opportunities for Fragile X. In these efforts, the NICHD is urged to collaborate with the three existing federally funded Fragile X Centers of Excellence as well as the Fragile X Clinics Consortium. The Committee requests the NICHD to report to Congress by September 1, 2008, on its progress in achieving these goals." (Senate Report 110-107, page 132).

Development of the Research Plan

Multiple steps were taken to develop the *Research Plan on Fragile X Syndrome and Associated Disorders*, as requested by the Senate Committee, in a manner that encouraged input from diverse sources. The first step was an outreach meeting convened in December 2007. Groups from the fragile X research community representing affected individuals and their families (FRAXA, NFXF) and the FXCC, along with other interested federal agencies in the DHHS, including the Centers for Disease Control and Prevention (CDC) and the Health Resources and Services Administration (HRSA), and in the Department of Education, were invited for the purpose of sharing current research activities and exploring possible opportunities to coordinate and collaborate in research efforts related to FXS and associated disorders.

The second step was to publish a Request for Information (RFI) in the NIH Guide for Grants and Contracts. *Research Priorities in Fragile X syndrome, Fragile X Tremor Ataxia syndrome, Premature Ovarian Failure and Other Relevant Conditions Associated with FMR1 Gene Function* was published in January 2008 cooperatively by the NICHD, the NIMH, the NINDS, the NIA, and the NIDDK and was distributed broadly throughout the scientific and fragile X advocacy community. The RFI sought input from the scientific community, health professionals, advocates, and industry related to future research priorities in the genetically related disorders of FXS, FXTAS, and FXPOI.

The third step was to establish three working groups of experts in the areas of FXS and the associated disorders of FXTAS and FXPOI to produce a plan of coordinated research strategies. The working groups included prominent researchers with diverse scientific expertise in areas such as psychology, genetics, epidemiology, neurology, genetic counseling, psychiatry, endocrinology, and molecular science. Most participating scientists had direct research experience in the area of FXS, FXTAS, or FXPOI, while others brought new research perspectives from fields focusing on similar or related disorders. The working groups also included clinicians who regularly treat individuals with FXS, FXTAS, and/or FXPOI. Advocates, parents, and participants from other interested federal agencies were also active and contributing members of the working groups. A chair was appointed to head each of the working groups. A roster of the working group members is included in this report, immediately following this section.

Charge to Working Groups

The charge to each working group was to identify priority areas of research to be used by the NIH and the FXS, FXTAS, and FXPOI research communities and shared with other federal agencies.

Each of the three working groups initially met via teleconference in March 2008. Through a series of teleconference calls and electronic communications, each working group developed a draft of specific goals and objectives. Working drafts of each working group's goals and objectives were available electronically, and members of the three working groups actively participated in developing, editing, and commenting on the documents.

In May 2008 the three working groups gathered in Bethesda, Maryland, for a two-day scientific meeting led by the NICHD and partners ORD, NIA, NINDS, and NIMH. The purpose of the meeting was to synthesize, fine-tune, and build upon drafts of goals and objectives developed by the working groups in the previous months. At the meeting each working group presented a draft of its goals to meeting participants. Discussion and constructive critiques from each of the three working groups and meeting participants led to further modification of the goals and objectives.

Subsequent to the two-day scientific meeting, each working group submitted a final draft of goals and objectives which NIH program and policy staff combined into a comprehensive research plan. The final draft report was submitted to each of the working groups for final editing and concurrence.

FXS and Associated Disorders Working Groups

FXS Working Group

Scientific and Constituency Group Participants (*DENOTES WORKING GROUP CHAIR)

*Don Bailey, Ph.D., Distinguished Fellow, RTI International

Leonard Abbeduto, Ph.D., Professor, Educational Psychology, University of Wisconsin–Madison

Elizabeth Berry-Kravis, M.D., Ph.D., Professor, Rush University Medical Center

W. Ted Brown, M.D., Ph.D., Director, New York State Institute for Basic Research in Developmental Disabilities

Katie Clapp, M.S., President/Cofounder, FRAXA–the Fragile X Research Foundation

William Greenough, Ph.D., Professor, University of Illinois at Urbana-Champaign

Randi Hagerman, M.D., Professor and Medical Director, M.I.N.D. Institute, University of California, Davis Health System

John March, M.D., M.P.H., Professor of Psychiatry and Chief of Child and Adolescent Psychiatry, Duke University Medical Center

Richard Paylor, Ph.D., Professor, Departments of Molecular and Human Genetics and Neuroscience, Baylor College of Medicine

Allan L. Reiss, M.D., Professor of Psychiatry and Director, Center for Interdisciplinary Brain Sciences Research, Department of Psychiatry and Behavioral Studies, Stanford University School of Medicine

Steven Warren, Ph.D., Chair, Department of Human Genetics, Emory University School of Medicine

Federal Participants

Judy Shanley, Ph.D., Education Program Specialist, Office of Special Education Programs, U.S. Department of Education

Julia Martin Eile, Ed.M., Education Program Specialist, U.S. Department of Education

Mark Swanson, M.D., Senior Medical Adviser, Department of Molecular Genetics and Microbiology, CDC

Carolyn Constantine, CDC

Marie Mann, M.D., M.P.H., Deputy Chief, Genetic Services Branch, HRSA

Cara Allen, Ph.D., Health Science Policy Analyst, NINDS

Richard Anderson, M.D., Ph.D., Program Director, NIGMS

Andrea Beckel-Mitchener, Ph.D., Chief, Functional Neurogenomics Program, NIMH

Lisa Gilotty, Ph.D., Chief, Social Behavior and Autism Program, NIMH

Robert Riddle, Ph.D., Program Director, Neurogenetics Cluster, NIMH

Tiina Urv, Ph.D., Health Scientist Administrator, NICHD

FXTAS Working Group
Scientific and Constituency Group Participants (*DENOTES WORKING GROUP CHAIR)

*Paul Hagerman, M.D., Ph.D., Professor and Director, NeuroTherapeutics Research, University of California, Davis

Tetsuo Ashizawa, M.D., Professor and Chairman of Neurology, University of Texas Medical Branch at Galveston

Elizabeth Berry-Kravis, M.D., Ph.D., Professor, Rush University Medical Center

Mary Beth Busby, FRAXA-the Fragile X Research Foundation

David Hessl, Ph.D., Assistant Professor, Department of Psychiatry and Behavioral Sciences, M.I.N.D. Institute, University of California, Davis

Peng Jin, Ph.D., Assistant Professor, the Department of Human Genetics, Emory University School of Medicine

Maureen LeeheyM.D., Professor of Neurology, University of Colorado at Denver and Health Sciences Center

David Nelson, Ph.D., Professor, Department of Molecular and Human Genetics, Co-director, Interdepartmental Program in Cell and Molecular Biology, Baylor College of Medicine

Maurice Swanson, Ph.D., Professor, University of Florida

Federal Participants

Pam Costa, M.A., Acting Director, National Center on Birth Defects and Developmental Disabilities, CDC

Robert Riddle, Ph.D., Program Director, Neurogenetics Cluster, NINDS

Stephen Snyder, Ph.D., Program Director, NIA

Tiina Urv, Ph.D., Health Scientist Administrator, NICHD

Karen Usdin, Ph.D., Senior Investigator, NIDDK

FXPOI Working Group
Scientific and Constituency Group Participants (*DENOTES WORKING GROUP CHAIR)

*Stephanie Sherman, Ph.D., Professor, Department of Human Genetics, Emory University

Mary Beth Busby, FRAXA (Fragile X Research Foundation)

Jodi Flaws, Ph.D., Professor, Epidemiology and Preventive Medicine, University of Illinois at Chicago

Gail Heyman, Parent Advocate, FRAXA-the Fragile X Research Foundation

Karima Hijane, Advocate, Rachel's Well

Corrine Kolka Welt, M.D., Assistant Professor of Medicine, Harvard University School of Medicine and Massachusetts General Hospital

Allyn McConkie-Rosell, Ph.D., CGC, Assistant Professor, Division of Medical Genetics, Department of Pediatrics, Duke University Medical Center

Kutluk Oktay, M.D., Professor and Section Chief, New York Medical College

Joe Leigh Simpson, M.D., Executive Associate Dean of Academic Affairs, Florida International University College of Medicine

Federal Participants

Joan Bailey-Wilson, Ph.D., Branch Chief, National Human Genome Research Institute, National Institutes of Health

Lawrence Nelson, M.D., Division of Intramural Research, NICHD

Natalie Street, Health Scientist, CDC

Susan Taymans, Ph.D., Program Director, NICHD

Tiina Urv, Ph.D., Health Scientist Administrator, NICHD

RESEARCH AREAS AND OBJECTIVES

In response to their charge the working groups developed a list of research priorities to guide future collaborative and directed efforts regarding FXS, FXTAS, and FXPOI. The goals are intended to be comprehensive (although not exhaustive) and include research priorities that extend from "bench-to-bedside-to-community." The goals were designed to be used by the NIH and the FXS, FXTAS, and FXPOI research communities and to be shared with other federal agencies to facilitate coordinated research activities that will lead to timely detection, diagnosis, treatment, and prevention of the targeted disorders.

The goals and objectives for each disorder are presented separately; this allows each section addressing a specific disorder to be part of the current document or to stand alone. While each disorder has unique research needs, there are some shared research themes that are discussed at the end of the *Research Areas and Objectives* section.

Each section (FXS, FXTAS, FXPOI) begins with a table summarizing research goals and objectives. The goals are listed in the table according to research theme and are presented in the order in which they appear in the plan. The working groups took care to balance the goals and objectives by the perceived risk in terms of success and the approximate time needed for achievment. Therefore, the objectives are categorized in the tables by: 1) the estimated time that it could take to accomplish them—short-term: zero to three years; intermediate-term: four to six years; or long-term: seven to ten years; and 2) the perceived risk in terms of success—low risk (LR), moderate risk (MR), high risk (HR). The working groups recognize that the perceived risk and time frames are subjective estimates and are only provided for guidance. The rationale for selecting goals and objectives and the impact of success on the field are described in each section.

The goals and objectives that follow are inspired by the current state of knowledge regarding each disorder. It is important to note that this knowledge remains incomplete, and therefore, the specific objectives recommended should not be interpreted to constrain creative research resulting from unforeseen novel discoveries.

FXS SUMMARY OF GOALS AND OBJECTIVES

Estimated time to accomplish goal: short-term (ST), zero to three years; intermediate-term (IT), four to sixyears; long-term (LT), seven to ten years.
Perceived risk in terms of success: low risk (LR), moderate risk (MR), high risk (HR).

Goal I - Advance Understanding of the Pathophysiology of FXS

Promote detailed examination of the molecular mechanisms *FMR1* gene and its mutations. Solidify understanding of the molecular mechanisms that lead to CGG repeat mutations and the consequences that alter *FMR1* gene expression, including modifications to or in regulatory and promoter regions as well as epigenetic modifications that lead to transcriptional silencing or modification (LT, MR).	Understand regulation of *FMR1* gene silencing and seek methods for targetable sequence-dependent restoration of expression. A first step in this regard is better models of gene silencing (LT, HR).	Work to create better models that more closely recapitulate the genetic instability and expansion mosaicism present in most cases of FXS (LT, MR).	Identify additional *FMR1* mutations in human populations and evaluate any functional variants that may inform pathophysiology and other phenotypes (IT, LR).	Delineate the cellular roles of FMRP and the macromolecules (mRNAs, microRNAs, proteins) with which it interacts (LT, IR).	Delineate the nervous system functional and structural phenotypes of FXS and of appropriate models (IT, MR).	Determine the impact of FXS and FMRP deficiency on neural systems. Investigate the mechanisms by which FMRP deficiency impacts synapses, plasticity, and connectivity (LT, MR).

Delineate the relationships(s) between behavioral abnormalities in animal models of FXS and underlying pathology and understand their relationship to the behavioral phenotype of individuals with FXS to ensure the use of optimal models of the disorder (LT, MR).

Goal II - Improve Appropriate and Timely Diagnosis of Individuals with FXS by Conducting Population-Based Screens

Develop and evaluate screening protocols to promote earlier identification of individuals with FXS in the broader population (ST, LR).	Develop and validate cost-effective and highly accurate laboratory tools for screening large numbers of individuals with all *FMR1* gene variations (IT, MR).	Evaluate the full range of costs and benefits of various approaches to population screening for FXS (LT, HR).	Determine the true incidence of *FMR1* gene variations and the extent to which the rate of these variants is consistent across major ethnic minority groups (IT, MR).

Goal III - Validate and Use Functional Measures of the Manifestation of FXS Across the Life Span

Develop a standard battery of functional, objective measures to better characterize the emergence of the FXS phenotype across the life span and provide precise indicators of treatment	Develop a standard battery of functional, objective measures to describe behavioral and psychosocial effects in *FMR1* premutation carriers across the life span and serve as indicators of treatment need and efficacy of treatment	Develop a biomarker discovery program of FXS, incorporating diverse technologies, approaches, and models to provide targets for treatment, accelerate the discovery of targeted pharmaceuticals, and	Conduct longitudinal studies of both humans and animal models to characterize the dynamic nature of the FXS phenotype across the life span and to identify moderators and mediators of the phenotype (LT,

effectiveness (ST, LR).	(IT, LR).	measure their efficacy (LT, MR).	MR).
		Develop effective interventions for individuals with the premutation who may experience developmental, psychosocial, and aging problems (LT, MR).	Leverage knowledge about biological pathways in FXS to design treatment studies for individuals with other developmental disabilities that share common pathophysiological mechanisms (LT, MR).
Goal IV - Initiate a Broad-Based Program of Research on the Efficacy of Treatments for FXS			
Evaluate and adapt current educational/behavioral interventions for individuals with the *FMR1* FXS and develop new interventions where indicated (IT, LR).	Pursue treatment targets that have shown promise in preclinical studies, including those for which drugs are currently in development and those for which approved drugs already exist, and carry out controlled trials of these drugs in adults and children with FXS as appropriate (IT, MR).	Understand the best timing of treatments and interventions across the life span for individuals with FXS (LT, MR).	
Goal V - Advance Understanding of the Ramifications of FXS for Families			
Conduct longitudinal research to more completely understand how families and family members adapt to FXS and related disorders (FXTAS, POI) and how adaptation changes over time and in response to developments within and external to the family (LT, LR).	Expand knowledge about how families from different cultures and ethnic minority groups interpret, respond to, and use information about FXS and the extent to which all families have equitable access to quality services (IT, LR).	Develop and evaluate the effectiveness of a wide range of supports for FXS families (LT, MR).	
Goal VI – Create a FXS Research Infrastructure and Resources to Maximize Research Efficiencies and Promote Large-Scale Research Collaboration			
Support and expand the availability of key research resources, from existing cellular-molecular level through digital imaging data (ST, LR).	Create new research resources and maximize their availability to the scientific community to enhance and accelerate understanding of biological and environmental effects on brain development and function associated with *FMR1* mutations (LT, MR).	Support of multisite research consortia and shared FXS databases to improve the efficiency and power of current and future research (LT, MR).	

FRAGILE X SYNDROME (FXS)

Goal 1 — Advance Understanding of the Pathophysiology of FXS

The most effective treatment for a complex disorder such as FXS is likely to emerge from a complete understanding of the anatomical, cellular, and molecular alterations that cause and result from the disorder. Treatments developed for other purposes, while possibly effective for aspects of the disorder, are unlikely to offer a complete substitute for the consequences of the absence of a gene product that likely modulates the expression of many other gene products. For this reason, understanding FXS at the genetic, molecular, cellular, nervous system, and behavioral levels is of vital importance to facilitate the development of rationally targeted treatments and more complete therapeutic interventions. Restated, it is through basic research into the biology of FXS that we are likely to develop insight into possibilities for effective therapeutic interventions.

Objective 1.1. Promote detailed examination of the FMR1 gene and its mutations. Solidify understanding of the molecular mechanisms that lead to CGG repeat mutations and the consequences that alter FMR1 gene expression, including modifications to or in regulatory and promoter regions as well as epigenetic modifications that lead to transcriptional silencing or modification.

Rationale. Nearly all known cases of FXS result from expansion of the CGG repeat in *FMR1* to sizes beyond ~230 triplets, a threshold above which the gene undergoes silencing due to chromatin alterations and methylation of the CGG repeats and the nearby promoter. Expansion from premutation-length repeats to the disease-causing full mutation requires female transmission. The mechanism of transition from premutation to full mutation has not been adequately defined, in part due to the absence of adequate animal models. Similarly, while much has been learned about the nature of the silenced *FMR1* locus in FXS, including detailed analysis of methylation and chromatin changes, the order and timing of events that lead to gene silencing remain incompletely understood.

Impact. Efforts to understand the aspects of repeat expansion and gene silencing that are unique to FXS have the potential to offer avenues to prevent or reverse them. The most likely effective characteristics of medicines will be those that restore, replace, or re-initiate normal chromatin regulatory functions. If the silencing of transcription of the *FMR1* gene could be selectively reversed in individuals with the disorder, it would be a major step towards restoring normal biological and behavioral functions in people with FXS.

Objective 1.2. Understand regulation of *FMR1* gene silencing and seek methods for targetable sequence-dependent restoration of expression. A first step in this regard is better models of gene silencing.

Rationale. A complementary, therapeutically oriented approach to Objective 1.1 would be to investigate the gene silencing by the *FMR1* full mutation with a goal to develop methods to restore expression. Work in this area has focused on both demethylating agents and compounds that alter chromatin methylation or acetylation. A potential approach to this problem would be to utilize a broader screen of agents using an appropriate assay for re-expression. Chemical libraries may be of use in such a screen. Alternatively, siRNA libraries, with each member able to suppress expression of each known human gene, may illuminate biochemical pathways controlling *FMR1* silencing and provide potential drug targets. A variation on this theme is the study of suppressed translation of *FMR1* mRNA carrying long CGG repeats. Some individuals with apparently full-mutation-length repeats have been observed to produce adequate amounts of FMRP—further study of the mechanistic aspects of this phenomenon, focused on translation, is warranted. Assays and chemical screens may also be of utility in understanding and potentially treating this aspect of gene silencing.

Impact. A targeted approach to the problem of *FMR1* gene silencing may offer new insights into the mechanism and point to possible treatment strategies.

Objective 1.3. Work to create better models that more closely recapitulate the genetic instability and expansion mosaicism present in most cases of FXS.

Rationale. Current mouse models do not adequately recapitulate this common *Fmr1* mutation. Loss-of-function (knockout [KO]) mice do not express full-length *Fmr1* at any time from their conception. This is in contrast to individuals with FXS, who often express *FMR1* in the majority of their cells early in development and in a fraction of their cells later in life due to the mosaic nature of the full mutation (mosaicism refers to a condition in which two or more cell populations differ in genetic makeup). Mice designed to carry expanded CGG repeats in the *Fmr1* gene have not adequately modeled the behavior of the human CGG triplets. Thus, improved models that offer animals that more closely mimic the human may prove advantageous. Alternatively, understanding the differences between the mouse and the human in triplet repeat behavior may offer mechanistic insight into the process in humans.

Impact. Improved animal models are essential to provide preclinical models of intervention. Current models are well suited to test treatment strategies for modifying complete loss of function but may not respond to therapy in a manner that will fully predict response by individuals with more complicated mosaic mutations. Improved models may also assist in understanding the impact of mosaic mutations and heterogeneity of CGG repeat length as well as the consequences of transcription/expression of full-mutation mRNA during early development (before methylation and silencing mechanisms).

Objective 1.4. Identify additional *FMR1* mutations in human populations and evaluate any functional variants that may inform pathophysiology and other phenotypes.

Rationale. Additional conventional mutations in individuals with aspects of FXS will provide significant insight into the functional domains of *FMR1* and consequences of alterations to gene and/or protein structure. A single missense mutation is known, along with numerous deletions and a small number of other loss-of-function mutations.

Impact. A concerted effort to identify individuals with fragile X mutations in *FMR1* would provide phenotype/genotype correlations and the potential to model these in experimental organisms.

Objective 1.5. Delineate the cellular roles of FMRP and of the macromolecules (mRNAs, microRNAs, proteins) with which it interacts.

Rationale. FMRP appears to operate in numerous cellular locations and may have multiple roles depending on the alternate splice variant isoform of FMRP, cell type, subcellular location, available binding partners, and/or posttranslational modification. This objective seeks to define the role(s) of FMRP in general, with emphasis on neuronal function in the presynaptic and postsynaptic compartments, cell body, dendrites, and in the nucleus. A key goal is to examine how FMRP operates in a synaptic activity-dependent manner to modulate plasticity in neurons. Current knowledge suggests a signal transduction pathway in dendrites that stems from signaling to Group 1 mGluRs that results in alterations in FMRP phosphorylation, mRNA translation, and AMPA (alpha-amino-3-hydroxy-5-methyl-4-isoxazoleproprionic acid) receptor internalization in the hippocampal mGluR5 long-term depression paradigm. It is likely that FMRP participates in other signaling pathways at other cellular locations, and these will be important to define. FMRP has been shown to control dendritic transport and modulate the translation of a large number of cargo mRNAs, including the mRNA for FMRP. Thus, a multiplicity of cellular effects result from its absence, and analysis of these effects may well suggest targets for drug intervention or replacement.

There are numerous avenues to approach FMRP function, many of which have received considerable attention to date. A number of these approaches are listed below. This is not meant to be an exhaustive list:

1.5.1. Characterize FMRP isoforms.

The *FMR1* gene expresses a significant number of alternatively spliced mRNA variants that produce numerous FMRP isoforms in all tissues studied. Whether these variant proteins have functional differences is unknown, but some are produced that lack key components for intermolecular interactions. Further efforts to characterize these isoforms for functional differences are recommended. It is noteworthy that many studies of FMRP function have relied on single isoforms introduced into cells or in protein assays. These studies may have missed significant features of alternative isoforms.

1.5.2. Develop assays for FMRP function.

Functional assays for FMRP have been challenging to develop. This is in part due to a lack of fundamental understanding of the protein's function but also due to its participation in a variety of activities involving other protein partners and target RNAs. Development of functional assays for FMRP and interacting (e.g., signaling) pathways would facilitate understanding of factors that contribute to FMRP function and allow the potential to screen for molecules that modify function. Currently, assays for FMRP function are best developed in intact animals, which are cumbersome for functional studies.

1.5.3. Characterize FMRP interactors.

Numerous protein partners have been identified, but the current list is unlikely to be complete. Among these are the paralogous proteins FXR1P and FXR2P, which are likely, based on similar amino acid sequence and structure, to carry out similar functions. Understanding their functions may lead to hypotheses regarding possible roles of FMRP. Moreover, these protein family members (FMRP, FXR1, and FXR2) can form complexes, and the consequences of absence of FMRP on the function(s) of these complexes will likely be informative from a basic science perspective and may prove to be relevant with regard to understanding FXS. In particular, the degree by which FXR1P and FXR2P may compensate in the nervous system for the loss of FMRP may be insightful. Other protein interactors include Cyfip1, Cyfip2 and Nufip, and analysis of their functions can similarly lead to better understanding of FMRP's role.

A significant body of evidence demonstrates the role of FMRP in mRNA metabolism, with likely roles in transport and control of local translation of a subset of cellular mRNAs. Efforts to define target RNAs have identified numerous candidates, with several showing significant alterations in models of the disorder. This catalog of target RNAs requires refinement, including additional validation of specific targets, in order to provide insight into pathways under the control of FMRP. Another key area that is incompletely understood is the role of microRNAs and the microRNA machinery in the mechanism of FMRP control of RNA location and translation. Investigation of these aspects of FMRP-mRNA interaction is also of particular interest.

1.5.4. Characterize FMRP's role in pathways.

The mGluR theory proposed to explain symptoms of FXS and findings in animal models of FMRP deficiency posits an overresponse to mGluR stimulation. In the mouse model of FMRP deficiency, evidence in favor of this theory is strong: both chemical and genetic reductions of mGluR5 can ameliorate phenotypes specific to *Fmr1* mutation. Similar evidence from chemical treatment of the fly model has been developed. Treatments based on reducing mGluR5 activation are currently being tested in patient populations. Continued follow-up on these observations at the human treatment level would seem to offer the best hope for the short-term development of effective treatments, with the caveat that, for unknown reasons, different brain regions have been shown to respond differently to mGluR5 drugs. Understanding the details of FMRP's participation in the pathway(s) leading from glutamate stimulation of Group 1 mGluR to phenotypes in model systems is a vital goal that will likely offer additional opportunities for intervention. It is also likely that FMRP participates in other signaling pathways at numerous cellular locations, and these will be important to define. For example, recent evidence from the fruit fly model of FXS points to GABA (gamma-aminobutyric acid) signaling as an interesting pathway to investigate, and electrophysiology studies suggest that muscarinic receptor signaling is altered in *Fmr1* KO mice, implying a broader involvement of G protein-coupled receptor systems.

1.5.5. Characterize FMRP's role in development.

It is frequently stated that FXS is a developmental disorder, in the sense that development is delayed and that delays are present from birth. There are also developmental anomalies in individuals that lead to some aspects of the physical phenotype. However, in a neuroanatomical sense, differences between the brains of individuals with FXS and typically developing individuals have been difficult to observe. Functional differences in cognition are clear, and it is currently not known what fraction of those differences stems from altered developmental trajectories and what comes from the acute absence of FMRP. Evidence from the fly model suggests that mGluR inhibitors can restore both functional and structural phenotypes late in development. The consequences of reintroduction of normally regulated levels of FMRP into a model that developed in the absence of FMRP are unknown. Studies of this type will help define the best outcome for treatment, and defining the developmental requirements for FMRP will also help to elucidate function.

Impact. FMRP, along with its interactors, appears to contribute to cell function by binding, transporting, and governing the local cellular translation of mRNA into the proteins it encodes. Whether that mechanism is related to the activity of mGluR5 receptors has not been determined. This research into G-protein-mediated cellular reactions, including mGluR5, may offer the best short-term approach for treatments of some of the most problematic behavioral symptoms, including aspects of autistic-like behavior. In the longer term, deficits in FXS likely involve failures in transport and localized translation. Replacement of either function of FMRP, or bypassing these functions to maintain appropriate cargo/target translation, could open the way to more effective therapeutic treatments.

Objective 1.6. Delineate the nervous system functional and structural phenotype of FXS and of appropriate models.

Rationale. Major advances in understanding FXS pathology have been made through characterization of models of FMRP deficiency in the mouse and fly. For example, the mGluR theory stemmed from the observation of subtle changes in long-term depression seen in the hippocampus of young *Fmr1* KO mice. Additional effort to define structural and functional phenotypes in models, along with further characterization of known phenotypes, is important to understanding pathology and potential areas of intervention in FXS. Improvement of existing models and development of novel models will be valuable. The recent development of conditional alleles of *Fmr1* in the mouse is one such example that will allow the investigation of the requirements for *Fmr1* in both time and location. Additional efforts in the fruit fly, zebrafish, and other models will also be useful. In this regard, cell-based and cell-free *in vitro* assays may also prove significant for defining neuronal function.

Impact. Models with well-defined phenotypes will assist with evaluation of treatments. Better understanding of the consequences of FMRP deficiency to the nervous system will also provide a wider variety of approaches to treatment.

Objective 1.7. Determine the impact of FXS and FMRP deficiency on neural systems. Investigate the mechanisms by which FMRP deficiency impacts synapses, plasticity, and connectivity.

Rationale. Initial findings of a difference in spine morphology and alterations in measures of plasticity in the nervous systems of FMRP-deficient mice have been encouraging. However, progress along other fundamental lines of inquiry with regard to brain phenotype has been slower than expected. Missing are fundamental data on cellular relationships ranging from the ultrastructure of synapses and neural tract studies to the consequences of neural architecture changes to behavior in both animal models and humans. There is a significant need to investigate these areas in patient samples and in a variety of models.

Impact. Understanding common consequences to neural systems will offer insight into the pathology of FXS and may provide additional avenues for potential amelioration of symptoms.

Objective 1.8. Delineate the relationship(s) between behavioral abnormalities in animal models of FXS and underlying pathology and understand their relationship to the behavioral phenotype of individuals with FXS to ensure the use of optimal models of the disorder.

Rationale. To fully utilize animal models, especially the *Fmr1* KO mouse model, it is essential to understand the molecular changes in the KO model that contribute to the behavioral abnormalities, but this relationship will best be optimized by fully understanding the nature of the behavioral abnormalities in *Fmr1* KO mice.

There are several behavioral abnormalities in the *Fmr1* KO mouse model that appear to be reliable across multiple laboratories. These traits represent the most powerful responses that can be utilized for understanding the relationship between abnormal behavioral responses in *Fmr1* KO mice and underlying molecular, morphological, and electrophysiological mediating events. Similarly, these behavioral abnormalities represent current traits that are optimal for identifying therapeutic interventions. However, the challenge in the field is the limited number of behavioral abnormalities that appear to be consistent with *a priori* expectations based on features of individuals with FXS. Findings such as increased activity, altered social interactions, increased sensitivity to audiogenic seizures, and some increased 'anxiety' in limited assays represent consistent behavioral abnormalities. However, there are several behavioral abnormalities that could be considered 'unexpected,' such as reduced acoustic startle, enhanced sensorimotor gating, and minimal impairments in learning and memory assays. There is a clear need to (a) better understand the nature of the behavioral abnormalities in *Fmr1* KO mice that are 'unexpected' and (b) identify and develop systematic tools to capture reliable cognitive impairments in *Fmr1* KO mice. It is essential to determine whether the unexpected behavioral findings in *Fmr1* KO mice are mediated by phenotypic characteristics similar to those found in individuals with FXS, and/or whether these represent inadequacies of the model or of the organism used to model the disorder.

Impact. Defining a role for FMRP deficiency in behavioral and cognitive impairments in animal models of FXS will be achieved by identifying robust assays that capture the appropriate impairments in animals lacking FMRP. Particular attention might be given to experiments focused on capturing FMRP-deficient learning and memory and other cognitive impairments. It is important for assays to be reliable across laboratories, to identify phenotypic differences that can be modulated by experimental interventions, and to require minimal specialized equipment. Exploration of other models of FXS, such as the *Fmr1* KO2 and I304N knock-in models, will assess their capacity to recapitulate behavioral and cognitive impairments observed in FXS. Lastly, consideration of developing a rat model for FXS that may be used to better to understand the role of FMRP deficiency in cognition is warranted, given the extensive literature on rat learning and behavior and its modification by psychoactive drug treatments.

The fragile X model in *Drosophila* has proven to be very useful for understanding the role of FMRP deficiency and abnormal behavioral responses associated with FXS. However, this model system is based on the *Drosophila* single FMRP/FXRP analog, which is not an exact parallel to FMRP in mammals. The fly model will doubtless continue to provide important insights into the relationship between FXS-related pathophysiology and behavior.

It is reasonable to begin to utilize mouse and fly models to screen for novel therapeutic interventions using *in vivo* behavioral endpoints that are robust and reliable across laboratories. In addition, both mouse and fly models may be used to identify and understand the role of modifier genes in regulating behavioral abnormalities in FXS.

Goal 2 — Improve Appropriate and Timely Diagnosis of Individuals with FXS by Conducting Population-Based Screening

FXS is still underdiagnosed, and many affected children are identified too late to maximize participation in early-intervention programs. Strategies are needed to increase physicians' awareness of FXS and promote early identification. Population-based screening is needed to determine the true prevalence of FXS within and across ethnic groups; assess the frequency of allele/carrier frequencies in the general population; create a more complete description of the full range of phenotypic expression (both primary consequences and secondary conditions); and further explicate the relationship between genotype and phenotype in both carriers and individuals with the full mutation. Screening studies would also be useful to understand the public's willingness to participate in screening for FXS status (both carrier and affected) at different life stages (preconception, prenatal, newborn, during childhood), and to understand the ways in which families and individuals adapt to and use genetic information obtained from screening.

Objective 2.1. Develop and evaluate screening protocols to promote earlier identification of individuals with FXS in the broader population.

Rationale. FXS has no physical features that are obvious at birth. Consequently, most individuals with FXS are identified after a family member becomes concerned about developmental or behavioral problems and a knowledgeable physician acknowledges these problems and specifically requests fragile X testing. For many families this process can take two to three years for males with the full mutation and much longer for females who typically demonstrate milder symptoms. Some children are identified much later and many may never be diagnosed, although the extent to which this occurs is unknown. As a result, many children miss the opportunity to benefit from early intervention programs, families experience costs and frustrations associated with their "diagnostic odyssey," and families make a range of decisions unaware of genetic risk for FXS. In the absence of newborn screening, other models for promoting earlier and broader identification of individuals with the full-mutation FXS need to be developed and evaluated. Various approaches that could be studied independently, or in combination, include increasing physicians' awareness of FXS, the incorporation in pediatric practice of routine developmental screening for all infants, developing and evaluating the usefulness of FXS-specific checklists, and prompt referral for genetic testing of any infant showing developmental delays. The ultimate goal would be to identify, evaluate, and implement comprehensive community-based practices to promote effective early identification of children with FXS.

Impact. Accomplishing this objective could reduce the age of identification of most children with FXS to 12 to 24 months. This would provide earlier access to early-intervention services and provide families with important information about their own genetic status and likelihood of additional children with FXS. Routine developmental screening in pediatric practice would also have positive ramifications for earlier identification of children who have or are at risk for other developmental disabilities.

Objective 2.2. Develop and validate cost-effective and highly accurate laboratory tools for screening large numbers of individuals with all *FMR1* gene variations.

Rationale. Currently, FXS syndrome is diagnosed using a combination of polymerase chain reaction (PCR) and Southern blot testing. These procedures are highly accurate for identifying individuals with the full mutation as well as premutation carriers, but the testing requires a blood sample and the cost ($250 to $400) is too great for large-scale research or screening. An inexpensive ($1 to $5) laboratory test would accelerate research to define the true incidence of *FMR1* gene variants, advance knowledge about the full range of genotype-phenotype correlations, and make possible broad-based public health screening. Ideally, such a test would be highly accurate, differentiate carriers from those with the full mutation, work equally well for males and females, and require only a small amount of blood (as in the case of blood spots on filter paper used for newborn screening) or other noninvasive biologic samples (e.g., saliva). The possibilities for useful applications will increase dramatically if FXS screening could be part of a platform that simultaneously tested for multiple conditions (as in the case of tandem mass spectrometry or oligonucleotide microarrays). Studies are needed to validate the accuracy of recently proposed screening methods, develop and evaluate alternative screening methodologies, and build capacity for rapid high-throughput screenng of large numbers of samples. An ultimate goal would be a multiplex platform that simultaneously screens for large numbers of conditions with great accuracy, low cost, and the capacity for large-sample testing.

Impact. The absence of a low-cost, accurate screening test is the primary impediment to more comprehensive identification of individuals with or at risk for FXS. Accomplishing this objective would make it possible to offer population-based screening and study the costs and benefits of offering screening at various ages. It would also facilitate large-scale research not currently possible, such as studies to determine the real incidence of FXS or the relationship between *FMR1* gene variations and various adverse health, emotional, or developmental outcomes. Studies such as these would be prohibitively expensive using current technology.

Objective 2.3. Evaluate the full range of costs and benefits of various approaches to population screening for FXS.

Rationale. Screening for FXS could be offered at different life stages — adults prior to conception, prenatal, newborn, during childhood. Currently, such screening is not routinely offered. For example, currently newborns in the United States are routinely screened for 20 to 55 conditions, depending on their state of residence. Conditions routinely screened for are primarily those for which an accurate and cost-effective screening test exists and for which an effective treatment exists that reduces morbidity and mortality associated with the disease.

FXS is not currently included in commonly used newborn screening panels because of the unavailability of an accurate, cost-effective screen and the lack of medical treatment for the disorder. However, recent developments are encouraging with regard to screening alternatives, and new medications may be more effective if started early in life. Detection of carrier status is an issue that needs to be considered when assessing the desirability of newborn screening for FXS. Additional issues arise if screening occurs at other times (e.g., prenatal screening), and these factors as well as others make FXS a good prototype for studying issues that will emerge in a new era of technological capabilities for genetic screening. Research is needed to understand the public's willingness to participate in screening for FXS status (both carrier and affected) at different life stages, how families and individuals adapt to and use genetic information obtained from screening, and the full range of costs and benefits of various forms and timing of screening.

Impact. The benefits and costs of screening, especially for carriers, are widely debated. Accomplishing this objective would provide critical information to help inform public policy and medical practice with regard to when, how, and whether screening for FXS can and should be offered on a population basis. Studies of screening for FXS would serve as a prototype for other genetic conditions and thus would be extremely informative in anticipation of technological advances that would make screening for many conditions possible.

Objective 2.4. Determine the true incidence of *FMR1* gene variations and the extent to which the rate of these variants is consistent across major ethnic minority groups.

Rationale. The true incidence of FXS is unknown. It is assumed that FXS occurs in almost every ethnic group and throughout the world, but some studies have suggested variability as a function of ethnic group or region of origin. However, samples have been far too small to provide definitive answers. Without this information, it is difficult to estimate the public health burden of FXS, whether rates of FXS are changing over time, or the extent to which some groups are at more or less risk for FXS than others. Population studies are needed to provide answers to these questions. Ideally these studies would be able to describe variations in allele frequencies as opposed to categorical reporting (e.g., full mutation, premutation, gray zone, normal). Data on gender and ethnicity would greatly add to this work, although race, ethnicity, and region of origin are increasingly complex constructs. Thus, research on cross-ethnic or cross-country variation will need to be conducted carefully to take such complexity into consideration when interpreting results. It is important that dissemination of findings on cross-ethnic variations be done with sensitivity to how these groups might interpret the results and that members of the groups studied should be included as stakeholders in designing an appropriate dissemination plan.

Impact. Accomplishing this objective would provide critical information about the real and potential public health burden of FXS. This information would enable a more accurate projection of the possible results and costs as well as be informative with regard to the evolutionary history of the *FMR1* gene. Better information on ethnic group variation could identify populations at greater or lesser risk and thus determine the extent to which ethnicity-related disparities exist in opportunities for diagnosis, treatment, and access to other necessary health care and services.

Goal 3 — Validate and Use Functional Measures of the Manifestations of FXS Across the Life Span

Many studies have documented a wide range of biological and behavioral effects of FXS. However, samples have been small and not population based. Symptoms associated with FXS (e.g., autism, anxiety, arousal, hyperactivity) have been measured in many different ways, with variable findings. Carriers have been understudied, and questions about whether and to what extent carriers are affected need to be addressed. There is no consensus on a core battery of behavioral and psychosocial assessments. A variety of physiological and neuroimaging techniques show promise and may be investigated further to determine their feasibility and validity. An intensive biomarker discovery program could help overcome these problems and could achieve these goals, particularly if it incorporates diverse technologies, methodological approaches, and models to provide targets for treatment, accelerate the discovery of targeted pharmaceuticals, and measure their efficacy. More research is needed to develop a standard battery of functional, objective measures to better assess phenotype and provide gold-standard indicators of treatment effectiveness.

Objective 3.1. Develop a standard battery of functional, objective measures to better characterize the emergence of the FXS phenotype across the life span and provide precise indicators of treatment effectiveness.

Rationale. There is little doubt that FXS is associated with effects on numerous dimensions of the phenotype, from the physical to the cognitive (e.g., executive function) and the social-affective (e.g., anxiety-related behaviors). The expression is variable across individuals, with some, especially females, displaying milder and more circumscribed effects and others displaying more severe and pervasive effects, including those leading to secondary diagnoses (e.g., autism). The current measures used to characterize the nature and severity of phenotypic effects, however, have been variable across studies and have involved small samples of participants. In addition, many of the measures used have poorly understood psychometric properties, have not been hypothesis driven, and have lacked precision (i.e., they often are influenced by many variables besides those of interest). The consequences of these measurement limitations are that the natural history of the disorder has not been fully characterized, the neurological underpinnings of many of the behavioral dimensions of the phenotype are unknown, and few phenotypic "targets" that could be used to measure treatment efficacy exist. Data are needed on a wide range of clinical symptoms associated with FXS, and studies of the relationship between FXS and other symptoms such as autistic behaviors or hyperactivity could increase understanding of both FXS and other clinically diagnosed conditions.

Impact. Accomplishing this objective would allow for a more complete understanding of the true nature and consequences of FXS. New measures could have applicability to a broad range of ages, degrees of affectedness, and range of contexts, from school to community and laboratory. Better measures would allow a more complete understanding of the relationships among measures at different levels of analysis, with the mapping of behavioral features onto underlying brain pathologies and onto biomarkers of the condition being especially important for understanding and treating the syndrome. This information could be used to evaluate the outcomes of various therapies, both pharmacological and educational, and to set the stage for development of FXS-specific environmental interventions that can optimize response to biological treatments.

Objective 3.2. Develop a standard battery of functional, objective measures to describe behavioral and psychosocial effects in *FMR1* premutation carriers across the life span and serve as indicators of treatment need and efficacy.

Rationale. Early assumptions that carriers of the *FMR1* premutation have no health effects have proven to be inacurate. Recent evidence has found that in some individuals the premutation is associated with serious health effects such as FXPOI in women and FXTAS, predominantly in aging men. There is also evidence of effects in the behavioral, neurocognitive, and psychosocial domains of individuals with the premutation who do not have FXPOI or FXTAS; however, these effects, if present, are more subtle and variable across studies, owing perhaps to a lack of robust measures for detecting effects and a reliance on small, nonrepresentative samples of participants. Recent findings using in-depth clinical interviews suggest that effects in the psychosocial realm may be of sufficient severity to warrant the provision of mental health services to a proportion of adult women who do not have FXPOI or FXTAS. As in the case of affected individuals with the full mutation, studies of premutation carriers may prove useful to focus on both core (i.e., condition-specific) features and co-occurring conditions and diagnoses (e.g., anxiety disorders, depression). These measures can be the foundation for research into the mechanisms producing the carrier phenotype and into the occurrence of the symptoms and conditions in the general population.

Impact. Accomplishing this objective would help determine to what extent premutation carriers experience challenges that adversely affect quality of life. Accomplishing this objective would also help identify the factors that moderate the expression of behavioral, neurocognitive, and psychosocial effects in carriers, with attention to both risk and protective factors. Ultimately, these may serve as outcome measures in tests of both drug and education/psychosocial interventions. Improving the physical and mental health of carriers would also have a positive impact on overall family function, including the outcome of children with FXS (i.e., full mutation).

Objective 3.3. Develop a biomarker discovery program of FXS, incorporating diverse technologies, approaches, and models, to provide targets for treatment, accelerate the discovery of targeted pharmaceuticals, and measure their efficacy.

Rationale. In recent years, a number of potential cell and molecular biomarkers that go beyond the genetic causes of FXS have been developed. These range from hormonal responses to stress to differences in the levels of some neurotransmitters and/or their receptors to differences in enzymatic and molecular phenomena that alter cellular metabolism and function. Examples include genotype-associated patterns of response to the neurotransmitter glutamate and alterations in enzyme pathways involved in cellular signaling. Considerable research remains to be conducted on these biomarkers. Indeed, many of the biomarkers available for human studies are crude (e.g., FMRP levels), although the science is more advanced in the development of biomarkers useful in other animal models. There is a need to determine empirically the relationships among these markers to determine if they organize themselves into clusters or constellations of biomarkers. In the case of human studies, this work is likely to involve physiological measures of CNS development and might include automated analysis of activity, movement, or facial expression, skin conductance, heart rate, event-related potentials, prepulse inhibition, MRI brain imaging techniques (anatomic magnetic resonance imaging [MRI], diffusion-tensor imaging [DTI], functional MRI [fMRI]), functional near-infrared spectroscopy (fNIRS), and positron emission tomography (PET) studies. In the case of nonhuman animal studies, this work will involve a wider range of variables, including neurotransmitters, enzymes, and other molecular measures. In studies of humans and other animals, it will be important to document how these measures differ from normal, to determine their consistency across species, and to find out how they relate to age-related changes and variability in individuals with FXS.

Impact. Accomplishing this objective would provide new information about treatment targets and could lead to the development of more effective pharmaceutical treatments. A more complete list of biomarkers and characterization of their responses to therapeutic drugs would position the field to identify the variables that might predict the efficacy and requisite dosage of new and traditional therapeutic drugs. These biomarkers could also be used to understand the biological systems that are affected in FXS and that mediate and moderate the expression of the phenotype.

Objective 3.4. Conduct longitudinal studies of both humans and animal models to characterize the dynamic nature of the FXS phenotype across the life span and to identify moderators and mediators of the phenotype.

Rationale. The identification of true "cause and effect" can be a difficult endeavor in human clinical research, and yet such information is crucial for developing more optimized interventions that address both genetic and environmental influences on outcome. Although investigators often make assumptions regarding etiology or pathophysiological mechanisms from cross-sectional research data, such assumptions are often later contradicted by longitudinal studies of the same clinical population. The manifestations of genetically influenced cognitive function or behaviors can be highly dynamic over development in the same individuals (or animals). Thus, there is a critical need for longitudinal studies to provide for more accurate phenotypic description for all *FMR1*-associated conditions. From a practical perspective, there is a need to understand the functional and adaptive abilities of individuals with FXS over time. Few data are available about early development and the precursors to later conditions (e.g., autistic behavior). Little is known about the nature of educational experiences, peer relations, physical and recreational activities, employment, or independent living for adults with FXS.

Impact. Accomplishing this objective could identify optimal times for intervention or prevention efforts, and it could provide additional insights into the mechanisms by which FXS affects functioning. It would also provide important information about the nature of support and age-appropriate services that would best meet the needs of individuals with FXS throughout the life span. Such information could also be used to develop early targeted interventions that prevent or at least decrease the severity of other conditions that may occur later in some individuals (e.g., self-injury).

Goal 4 — Initiate a Broad-Based Program of Research on the Efficacy of Treatments for FXS

Although many studies have focused on the nature and consequences of FXS, there is a dearth of research on the efficacy of treatments. A few studies have examined the efficacy of traditional medications (e.g., stimulants) in humans, and recent early-stage trials have begun using more targeted treatments. Promising studies in the past two years have shown significant treatment effects of targeted medications, such as mGluR antagonists, in selected nonhuman models. Virtually no research has been conducted on the efficacy of educational, psychological, or therapeutic interventions in FXS. Major work is needed to study the efficacy of a wide range of treatment options, both known and emerging, in both animal and human models. This research may combine disease-specific knowledge about FXS with more general knowledge about effective interventions derived from studies of other conditions. Research is needed not only on individual treatments but also on the effectiveness of combinations of treatments, including the integration of targeted pharmaceutical treatments with optimization of the social and educational environment to maximize learning and adaptation.

Objective 4.1. Evaluate and adapt current educational/behavioral interventions for individuals with FXS and develop new interventions where indicated.

Rationale. Animal models have demonstrated that an enriched environment can normalize the synaptic structure in the *Fmr1* null mouse. There have been few studies to assess the efficacy of educational or behavioral interventions in individuals diagnosed with FXS. The behavioral interventions used for autism have not widely been tested in individuals with FXS diagnosed either with or without autism. Controlled studies may be useful in assessing the effects of a range of behavioral and educational interventions, including those that make use of assistive technology devices. These issues become particularly important if targeted pharmaceutical or other biological treatments for FXS can make synaptic connections more receptive to environmental interventions. This research is an exciting endeavor both for adults with FXS who may now be able to learn from a lifetime of education and for children whose development can be more normalized. Effective supports and services for adults with FXS need to be identified to maximize independence, peer socialization, physical health, and adaptive living. In addition, cutting-edge educational interventions, such as the use of virtual-reality paradigms, may be fruitful areas of study.

Impact. This research could significantly change the way that education and support services are provided for both children and adults with FXS. Demonstrating the efficacy of a wide range of educational, psychological, therapeutic, and other functional interventions could enhance the speed with which they are incorporated into birth-to-three services, the public school curriculum, or adult supports and services. These interventions can also be implemented in conjunction with medical interventions, and their relative and combined efficacy may be studied.

Objective 4.2. Pursue treatment targets that have shown promise in preclinical studies, including those for which drugs are currently in development and those for which approved drugs already exist, and carry out controlled trials of these drugs in adults and children with FXS as appropriate.

Rationale. Trials of medications such as mGluR5 antagonists, including MPEP (2-methyl-6-[phenylethynyl]pyridine), fenobam, and other compounds, have been carried out in various animal models of FXS, including the *Fmr1* null mouse model, the *Drosophila dfmr1*-null model, and even the zebrafish model, demonstrating evidence of efficacy in improving learning, seizures, and some behavior. Fenobam has recently been identified as an mGluR5 antagonist. Toxicity studies have now been carried out, and controlled trials can be initiated regarding fenobam in adults and subsequently children with FXS. Other mGluR5 antagonists have been developed and are also close to human studies. The stress pathway (hypothalic-pituitary-adrenal axis) and cholinergic brain systems also appear to be important in the pathogenesis of cognitive and behavioral dysfunction in animal models and human FXS. As with the mGluR compounds, trials are under way to "normalize" function of these systems in FXS with already available pharmacological agents. Numerous additional potential drug targets have also been suggested, based upon animal models of FXS. Thus, multiple potential drug targets may exist, and there is a need for simple cellular or protein-based assays that mimic abnormalities in FXS that could be used for small molecular screening of chemical libraries.

Impact. The development of effective disease-specific treatments would have a dramatic impact on the clinical condition of FXS, leading to improved behavior and learning. This would be tremendously helpful for individuals and families who struggle on a daily basis with their children, and it would dramatically improve the functioning of these individuals, including their long-term prognosis and integration into society.

Objective 4.3. Understand the best timing of treatments and interventions across the life span for individuals with FXS.

Rationale. Human and animal studies to date have not yet determined how effective specific treatments and interventions for FXS may be across the life span — the newborn period, childhood, adolescence, and adulthood. Critical periods in development may limit the usefulness of certain specific treatments to childhood. As more-specific treatments are explored, it becomes increasingly important to understand when these treatments might be useful so as to design appropriate animal and human trials. If newborn screening becomes a reality, many more babies will be identified, providing the opportunity to conduct research to evaluate the most effective intervention paradigms for babies. Information regarding how infants process information can help to shape new intervention techniques. Ultimately, to be most effective new medical interventions may need to be provided early in life, but this assumption will need rigorous testing. The development of new intervention programs may be beneficial to a larger population of children with developmental delays.

Impact. These studies could significantly improve treatment at all ages from newborns to old age. Although the emphasis currently is on treatment in children, studies throughout the age span will improve the interventions offered to adults. In addition to treatment protocols, preventive interventions could help avoid future problems.

Objective 4.4. Develop effective interventions for individuals with the *FMR1* premutation who may experience developmental, psychosocial, and aging problems.

Rationale. A subgroup of individuals with the *FMR1* premutation may experience physical, developmental, or psychosocial problems that interfere with function and/or quality of life. There is a need to better understand the nature and consequences of effects experienced by carriers and to identify which individuals are most vulnerable to developmental problems either from lowered FMRP levels, elevated mRNA levels, or other additive factors to these molecular changes. The pathophysiology of developmental problems could be studied along with interventions that might be efficacious in childhood to prevent the later onset of possible problems. Effective counseling and other support strategies need to be studied in order to promote positive psychosocial adaptation of carriers.

Impact. FMR1 premutation carriers not only experience the burden of their reproductive risk status but may also experience problems in health and development and lower quality of life. Identifying the carriers who are at risk for these problems and intervening early could enhance the lives of these individuals, their children, and their families. Prophylactic intervention for FXTAS or related conditions could significantly increase the productive lifetime and quality of life for carriers.

Objective 4.5. Leverage knowledge about biological pathways in FXS to design treatment studies for individuals with other developmental disabilities that share common pathophysiological mechanisms.

Rationale. Many individuals with FXS experience other conditions such as attention deficits, anxiety, aggression, hyperactivity, and seizure disorders, and they may also meet the diagnostic criteria for autism. Multiple lines of study suggest that overlapping pathways are affected in several developmental disorders. If this is the case, treatments being developed for FXS might effectively treat many other patient populations, and vice versa.

Impact. Developing and evaluating the efficacy of treatments for FXS could have implications for improving function in some individuals with autism or other conditions, especially those with shared symptoms (such as attention-related problems), and individuals with FXS and carriers may benefit from knowledge gained from other disorders. Sharing knowledge and increasing opportunities for dialogue between different communities of researchers and would be beneficial to all.

Goal 5 — Advance Understanding of the Ramifications of FXS for Families

Families of individuals with FXS, like families of all children with disabilities, must help their children learn functional skills, develop social competence, and regulate or control challenging behaviors. But FXS poses unique issues for families. Families need to inform siblings and their own parents and often feel obligated to encourage relatives to obtain genetic testing. Families may deal with guilt for having transmitted a disorder to their child. They must decide when and how to tell carrier children about their reproductive risk status. Carriers may also be at risk for social, emotional, and other challenges by virtue of carrying the premutation, they may feel stigmatized, and their reproductive risk status may affect their ability to establish and maintain relationships. Some mothers have the full mutation themselves and may face challenges in their capacity to care for their children. Research is needed to develop a deeper understanding of the family consequences of FXS at the level of the individual as well as at the level of the family, and to identify the types of supports needed to promote positive adaptation.

Objective 5.1. Conduct longitudinal research to more completely understand how families and family members adapt to FXS and related syndromes (FXTAS, FXPOI) and how adaptation changes over time and in response to developments within and external to the family.

Rationale. Research on family adaptation to FXS has almost exclusively focused on maternal adaptation. Continued research on mothers is needed, but little is known about how fathers, siblings, grandparents, and other extended family members adapt to information about FXS, despite the inevitable ramifications for extended family members. More needs to be known about communication patterns within families and whether or how family relationships change as a result of FXS, FXTAS, or FXPOI. Little is known about how families cope with fragile X across the life span, especially as children become adults and families adjust to changing patterns of services, residential accommodations, and aging. It may prove valuable to examine a range of outcomes, including the challenging consequences of FXS as well as the ways families have used FXS to enhance their lives. Full understanding of family adaptation will likely require a mixture of quantitative and qualitative research to understand how families are affected by FXS as well as how families in turn can influence the characteristics and level of functioning of individuals with FXS.

Impact. Accomplishing this objective would provide important insights into the complicated ramifications of FXS for families and the various strategies that families use to adapt successfully. The identification of factors associated with successful adaptation could lead to the development of effective supports and interventions for families, including those that can prevent or at least lessen later negative outcomes that might otherwise occur.

Objective 5.2. Expand knowledge about how families from different cultures and ethnic minority groups interpret, respond to, and use information about FXS and the extent to which all families have equitable access to quality services.

Rationale. Virtually nothing is known about FXS in families from ethnic minority groups and low-resource families. It is widely thought that FXS is underdiagnosed in ethnic minority groups. Research with other genetic conditions suggests that some people are uncertain about the value of genetic information or are concerned about potential stigmatization of groups. Different cultures have different family structures and patterns of support. It is unknown how families from diverse cultures would respond to population-based screening programs for FXS. Substantial research is needed in this area. A short-term objective would be to conduct small descriptive studies of families from diverse cultures. Ultimately, however, such studies would need much larger samples and more diverse populations. This, in turn, would require a cost-effective screening test and a concentrated effort to assure the acceptability of genetic information to diverse cultures.

Impact. Accomplishing this objective would help to put in place the tools and knowledge needed to promote access to diagnosis and quality services for all families and would provide important information about ways to provide culturally sensitive genetic counseling and family support services.

Objective 5.3. Develop and evaluate the effectiveness of a wide range of supports for FXS families.

Rationale. Despite the challenges experienced by families with FXS, little research has systematically evaluated the efficacy of various approaches to and models for the provision of services, such as genetic counseling, family support, general and mental health, or enhanced parenting skills. A broad-based program of treatment research is needed to enhance understanding among families about FXS; maximize the quality of the home environment; and help families deal with the learning, behavioral, and emotional challenges they face. A near-term objective would be to evaluate the efficacy of known family support programs (e.g., training in parenting, parent-to-parent support groups) that have been developed for families of children with other disabilities. A longer-term objective would be the development and evaluation of strategies that are unique to supporting families with FXS.

Impact. FXS has widespread ramifications for families, but little is available in terms of systematic support for families. Accomplishing this objective would identify evidence-based practices to support families.

Goal 6 — Create a FXS Research Infrastructure and Resources to Maximize Research Efficiencies and Promote Large-Scale Research Collaboration

Most research in FXS to date has relied on individual investigator-initiated efforts, with little in the way of broad infrastructure support. While this might have been sufficient in the early stages of research, the field has made sufficient advances so that specific core supports would now enhance the quality, timeliness, and efficiency of research. Four examples of areas of needed infrastructure are: (1) a broader array of appropriate nonhuman models of FXS easily accessible by researchers from a variety of institutions; (2) a human brain and tissue bank; (3) better, standardized and more widely available research reagents (e.g., antibodies) and experimental compounds for preclinical studies; and (4) a patient registry or research consortium to maximize access to a large number of individuals with FXS for both descriptive and intervention studies.

Objective 6.1. Support and expand the availability of key research resources, from the existing cellular-molecular level through digital imaging data.

Rationale. At this time, the field is sufficiently mature to offer a number of key resources that cross multiple scientific levels of investigation. For example, the original *Fmr1* null mouse is available on several genetic backgrounds, as are cell lines for various FXS- related conditions.

The *Drosophila* model system is also available for study and increasingly used by investigators. For example at the tissue or brain bank level, there are relatively fewer resources available, and these are not widely publicized. Augmented support is needed to enhance the availability and distribution of current resources such as animal models (e.g., mice, *Drosophila*), brain, and other tissue cell lines, including stem cells.

Impact. Greater availability of key research resources will permit larger numbers of investigators to test important hypotheses and replicate previous findings related to *FMR1* mutation-related disorders. Greater resource availability and larger samples will also allow for more robust study results with greater validity.

Objective 6.2. Create new research resources and maximize their availability to the scientific community to enhance and accelerate understanding of biological and environmental effects on brain development and function associated with *FMR1* mutations.

Rationale. Current animal models have been very useful in developing and testing hypotheses related to human FXS. However, new models (Objective 1.3) and biological samples are needed to augment and enhance this work. In addition to animal models and biological tissues, digital data such as those acquired from human or animal imaging studies will be of potential benefit, particularly as related to future treatment studies that will rely on in vivo serial imaging to follow or predict treatment effects. Specific examples of needed resources include: (1) new KO and transgenic mice (e.g., I304N KI, YAC Tg298, various CGG repeat expansion mice, and KO mice for Fxr1/2); (2) new model systems, in addition to *Drosophila*, with emphasis on viable conditional KOs; (3) improved reagents, including monoclonal antibodies; and (4) imaging data banks from animal and human studies including MRI, PET, and gene expression imaging.

Impact. New animal models, tissue samples, and digital databases will allow investigators to develop and test new hypotheses directly related to the identification, pathogenesis, and treatment of *FMR1* mutation-related disorders. These advanced research resources will usher in the next generation of basic and clinical research studies in this area.

Objective 6.3. Support of multisite research consortia and shared FXS databases to improve the efficiency and power of current and future research.

Rationale. Enhancing inter-institution collaboration for multisite and multidisciplinary studies and shared databases provides clear-cut advantages for advancing research, particularly for rare disorders. In the short term, important activities would include: (1) the development of a Web site that describes ongoing fragile X-related human research projects and clinical trials similar to that implemented at NCI; (2) investigator meetings focused on data sharing, registries, and the development of new interdisciplinary and cross-disciplinary research consortia; and (3) expanded ways to include subjects with FXS in clinical trials, including trials for other disorders such as autism. It would be valuable for private and public agency personnel to meet with lead investigators to discuss collaborative research, including private-public partnerships, policies about data sharing, and collaborative and multidisciplinary/interdisciplinary research proposals. A multisite clinical research consortium (e.g., the existing FXCC) is needed to test new FXS-specific treatments based on rapidly expanding knowledge of disease pathophysiology. These clinics would be prepared to use standardized methods for assessment and treatment, thus maximizing subject numbers and representation from the general population.

Impact. As shown in other research fields, the benefits to enhancing organization and infrastructure to facilitate data sharing and research collaboration include the ability to recruit larger numbers of more representative subjects for research studies and the standardization of clinical trials relative to assessment and/or treatment methods, the collection and availability of significantly larger samples of biological samples or digital data, cross-fertilization of ideas across investigators and institutions and, eventually, new and improved state-of-the-art practice parameters to improve outcome in affected individuals with disease-specific interventions. For *FMR1* mutation-related disorders, such benefits may be even more tangible, as the field stands on the brink of developing and testing new therapies that directly address disease pathogenesis.

FXTAS SUMMARY OF GOALS AND OBJECTIVES

Estimated time to accomplish goal: short-term (ST), zero to three years; intermediate-term (IT), four to six years, long-term (LT), seven to ten years.
Perceived risk in terms of success: low risk (LR), moderate risk (MR), high risk (HR).

Goal I – Defining Pathogenic Mechanisms of FXTAS

Define the specific molecular mechanisms (e.g., expanded CGG-repeat *FMR1* mRNA) that initiate downstream events leading to FXTAS pathology (IT, LR).	Define the mechanisms leading to overexpression of the expanded CGG-repeat mRNA (IT, LR).	Identify the molecular basis for incomplete penetrance of FXTAS, including gender-specific differences in penetrance and the extent to which penetrance reflects second-gene effects and/or environmental factors (LT, HR).	Determine the mechanism of formation and pathogenic significance of the intranuclear inclusions of FXTAS (IT, MR).	Understand the pathogenic basis for the significant white matter disease present in FXTAS (IT, MR).	Define the programmed cell-death mechanism(s) (e.g., apotosis or paraptosis) that are operating in FXTAS (IT, MR).	Establish additional animal models (e.g., invertebrate, mouse, primate, other) to study pathogenic mechanisms of FXTAS (e.g., mice with inducible and conditional expression of the CGG repeat in various reporter contexts, or primate models of FXTAS, which will display the behavioral and cognitive phenotypes that are more similar to the human clinical phenotypes) (IT, MR).

Goal II – Defining FXTAS Clinical Phenotypes

Define the broader range of neurological, neurocognitive, behavioral, and emotional dysfunction associated with FXTAS (ST, LR).	Develop and validate instruments that quantify clinical signs, including motor and neuropsychological signs, and progression of disease and instruments that are sensitive to early signs of FXTAS progression; identify the most sensitive and predictive parameters to include in these instruments through clinimetric testing (ST, LR).	Identify molecular, clinical, and environmental risk and protective factors associated with the penetrance of FXTAS (IT, MR).	Prospectively identify the natural history of the *FMR1* premutation carrier and FXTAS progression, including factors associated with rapid and slow progression of disease (IT, MR).	Define the relationship between the FXTAS clinical phenotype, *FMR1* molecular genetic abnormalities, imaging, and measures of cellular pathology; identify factors (e.g., molecular, clinical, environmental) associated with various FXTAS clinical signs (IT, MR).

Goal III – Epidemiology of FXTAS and *FMR1* Premutation Alleles

Define the prevalence of the *FMR1* allele lengths in the general population	Determine the prevalence of elongated *FMR1* alleles in adults with genetically	Identify potential familial predisposition to FXTAS, its association with FXPOI

ascertained in an unbiased fashion. Categorize these data for age; data across numerous age cohorts is desirable (IT, LR).	undefined movement disorders (e.g., ataxia, tremor, parkinsonism), memory impairment or dementia (e.g., Lewy body dementias, Alzheimer disease), dysautonomia, and/or peripheral neuropathy (IT, LR).	and FXS, and find molecular factors involved in family clustering (IT, LR).

Goal IV – Early Diagnosis/Identification of Individuals Most At Risk of Developing FXTAS

Develop molecular markers of cellular toxicity (e.g., metabolic, regulatory) that are assayable in a peripheral tissue or fluid of individual carriers to assist with prediction of impending disease before symptoms develop, finding those most at risk, and tracking cellular toxicity in carriers, with age, and after interventions (IT, HR).	Develop radiological markers of CNS toxicity through more sensitive measures, such as DTI or MR spectroscopy (MR-SPECT), that will indicate individuals at risk for FXTAS before clinical symptoms or standard radiological signs of FXTAS become evident (LT, LR).	Use the cellular, radiological, and clinical markers associated with FXTAS to successfully track improvements in toxicity measures with preventative or symptomatic treatment in clinical trials (LT, HR).
Utilize theser markers to assist with drug discovery for targeted treatments that block the mechanism of toxicity in the underlying disorder (LT, HR).		

Goal V – Supportive and Targeted Therapeutic Interventions for FXTAS

Evaluate currently available pharmaceutical treatments targeted at specific symptoms in FXTAS to determine if they are helpful in well-designed clinical trials. Examples would be memantine for neurodegeneration and cognitive decline, minocycline and other putative neuroprotective agents, and standard treatments targeted at reduction of tremor (ST, LR).	Evaluate existing supportive devices and physical therapies to determine if these improve outcome (e.g., increase time to becoming wheelchair bound) or lengthen survival of persons with FXTAS (ST, LR).	Evaluate new drugs currently in development (e.g., oxybate, mGluR5 blockers) that are targeted to FXTAS symptoms in trials in animal models and human clinical trials (IR, MR).	Utilize screening techniques that test the effect of large numbers of medications in cell culture and in animal models in reducing the toxic mechanisms that occur in FXTAS (IT, HR).
			Evaluate novel therapeutic agents (e.g., RNAi, proteins or peptides, other small molecules) that may reverse cellular toxicity and may reverse or prevent FXTAS symptoms in animal models and in human clinical trials aimed at both treatment and prevention (LT, HR).

Goal VI – Quality-of-Life Issues Associated with FXTAS

Assess the attitudes of individuals and their families about receiving a *FMR1* premutation diagnosis, the optimum time to receive this information, and their interest level regarding learning their carrier status to determine how much information may be shared with parents when a child is identified as being a carrier and who in the family needs to know (ST, LR).	Determine the availability and adequacy of genetic counseling for families, its usefulness and complexity, and the understandability of information provided through counseling after diagnosis as an *FMR1* premutation carrier (ST, LR).	Determine the impact of the *FMR1* premutation carrier diagnosis on the quality of life of the carrier individual and of other family members and design interventions to reduce the negative effects on quality of life (IT, MR).	Determine whether quality of life for those affected with FXTAS and their family members is most affected by motor, psychological/psychiatric, or cognitive dysfunction in the individual with FXTAS and determine which aspects of the quality of life are most affected (ST, LR).	Develop, implement, and evaluate supportive interventions for individuals with FXTAS and their families (LT, HR).	Determine the level of awareness among FXTAS-affected families regarding support systems at fragile X clinics and resource groups and their perception of need, adequacy, and availability of expertise in neurological management, psychological/counseling support, and availability of information on possible treatment options (IT, LR).

Goal VII – Broader Implications for other Neurodegenerative Diseases

Identify the disease pathways that are shared by FXTAS and more common neurodegenerative disorders, such as idiopathic Parkinson disease and Alzheimer disease (LT, MR).	Determine the extent to which Parkinson disease-associated mechanisms (e.g., problems with the cell's ability to dispose of abnormally folded proteins, dysfunction of the energy-producing mitochondria, and oxidative damage) also play roles in FXTAS pathogenesis (IT, MR).	Determine whether the premutation influences the course of other neurodegenerative or non-CNS diseases (IT, MR).	Develop conditional/inducible animal models that recapitulate specific neurotoxic events common to FXTAS and other neurodegenerative diseases (LT, HR).	Establish research initiatives and forums that promote collaborations between investigators studying FXTAS and other late-onset neurodegenerative disorders (LT, LR).

Goal VIII – Establishing a General Research Infrastructure for FXTAS

Clinical	Establish standardized endpoints for preclinical trials in animal models and ensure that facilities are available that enable testing of drugs and other therapeutic approaches (LT, LR).	Create a mechanism to maintain animal (e.g., mouse) models of FXTAS at approved vendors in a live state that are available for easy and rapid importation into academic colonies (MT, LR).	Encourage the development of cell-based assays (e.g., stem cell-based technologies) that target aspects of pathogenesis and pathophysiology in FXTAS (MT, HR).	
Clinical Research and Trial Infrastructure	Establish a *FMR1* premutation patient registry and clinical data and	Develop a consortium of clinics to work with individuals with FXTAS,	Monitor, coordinate, and communicate the rehabilitation and	

	sample repositories, including DNA, cells, and tissues (IT, LR).	where there would be expertise in the use of optimal outcome measures and through which clinical trials could be run at multiple sites in a standardized fashion for future multicenter trials (LT, LR).	educational assessment activities of the various federal agencies and voluntary and advocacy groups (LT, LR).
Communication and Education	Design and implement a Web site that provides information and links to all existing FXTAS resources in both the United States and internationally (ST, LR).	Stimulate international collaborations and infrastructure sharing to ensure that opportunities in FXTAS research are exploited and resources are used to maximum advantage (ST, IR).	

FRAGILE X-ASSOCIATED TREMOR/ATAXIA SYNDROME (FXTAS)

Goal 1 — Defining Pathogenic Mechanisms of FXTAS

FXTAS is a neurodegenerative disorder that results from the abnormal expression of moderately expanded (premutation) forms of the *FMR1* gene. A more detailed understanding of the consequences of this abnormal expression is likely to yield targeted (disease-specific) therapeutic approaches for FXTAS. Furthermore, because downstream events in FXTAS neurodegeneration are likely to at least partially overlap those of other neurodegenerative disorders (e.g., Parkinson and Alzheimer diseases), defining the pathogenic mechanisms of FXTAS may yield therapeutic approaches that could be more generally applied to the more common neurodegenerative disorders.

Research in FXTAS will provide a unique opportunity to develop a class of disease-targeted therapeutic agents because the fundamental triggering events are reasonably well understood. Because the cellular dysregulation and death mechanisms are likely to, at least partially, overlap the mechanisms associated with the major neurodegenerative disorders, the therapeutic agents developed for FXTAS would be expected to have broader therapeutic applicability.

Objective 1.1. Define the specific molecular mechanisms (e.g., expanded CGG-repeat *FMR1* mRNA) that initiate downstream events leading to FXTAS pathology.

Rationale. Unlike many other sporadic neurodegenerative disorders, FXTAS has a clearly defined genetic mutation, which provides greater opportunity to dissect the pathogenic mechanism and to define key elements in the degenerative pathway that would serve as targets for therapeutic intervention.

Impact. Understanding the regulatory mechanisms of CGG expansion and the initial pathogenic pathway immediately downstream of the gene mutation would guide the development of strategies for FXTAS-specific therapeutic interventions, which are expected to be more effective than interventions in the more indirect pathways.

Objective 1.2. Define the mechanisms leading to overexpression of the expanded CGG-repeat mRNA.

Rationale. The reasons why carriers of the FXS premutation show overexpression of the *FMR1* mRNA are not understood. Because RNA toxicity appears to be the dominant pathogenic trigger, research to understand the regulation of *FMR1* mRNA expression may lead to the development of interventions that reduce expression below toxic levels.

Impact. Identification of the mechanism by which the *FMR1* gene overexpresses its mRNA will have general scientific impact for other genes where the CGG repeat may lead to toxicity and will serve as a basis for designing therapeutic approaches to treat FXTAS.

Objective 1.3. Identify the molecular basis for incomplete penetrance of FXTAS, including gender-specific differences in penetrance, and the extent to which penetrance reflects second-gene effects and/or environmental factors.

Rationale. The molecular basis of reduced penetrance and the gender dependency of the reduced penetrance are unknown. However, acquiring this knowledge is important both for identifying who is at risk and for determining whether there are any protective factors involved with non-penetrance.

Impact. Accomplishing this objective will provide an explanation for the complex genotype-phenotype correlation in FXTAS; understanding why some individuals remain non-penetrant may also lead to development of rational treatments for FXTAS.

Objective 1.4. Determine the mechanism of formation and pathogenic significance of the intranuclear inclusions of FXTAS.

Rationale. The mechanism of formation and pathogenic role of the intranuclear inclusions in FXTAS is unknown.

Impact. Intracellular inclusions are a hallmark of many neurodegenerative diseases, and understanding the mechanism(s) of formation and the pathogenic significance of FXTAS inclusions may reveal the functional significance of the formation of inclusions in other neurodegenerative diseases.

Objective 1.5. Understand the pathogenic basis for the significant white-matter disease present in FXTAS.

Rationale. White-matter disease is a prominent finding in FXTAS. However, the pathogenic basis for the white-matter disease is poorly understood. Identification of the causes of this brain pathology and when it develops may lead to chances of early intervention before there is substantial loss of neurons in the CNS.

Impact. An understanding of the factors leading to white-matter disease in FXTAS, including those interventions that may specifically reduce the extent of damage, may lead to both better prognosis and additional therapeutic targets for this disorder. Moreover, because features of the white-matter pathology in FXTAS are shared with other neurodegenerative disorders, lessons learned through the study of this pathology will have broader impact on therapeutic interventions in other neurodegenerative disorders.

Objective 1.6. Define the programmed cell-death mechanism(s) (e.g., apoptosis or paraptosis) that are operating in FXTAS.

Rationale. There are a small number of cell-death mechanisms that represent the outcomes of the pathogenic processes in neurodegeneration; such mechanisms are common to many neurodegenerative diseases, although their triggers and pathways are generally poorly understood. Because its pathogenic trigger (RNA toxicity) is known, FXTAS represents an important model for the study of neurodegeneration.

Impact. Understanding the cell-death mechanism in FXTAS may provide additional details of cell-death mechanisms operating in other neurodegenerative diseases. These same models may facilitate the development of preventative approaches as well as therapeutic measures.

Intrastructure Needs
Objective 1.7. Establish additional animal models (e.g., invertebrate, mouse, primate, other) to study pathogenetic mechanisms of FXTAS (e.g., mice with inducible and conditional expression of the CGG repeat in various reporter contexts, or primate models of FXTAS, which will display the behavioral and cognitive phenotypes that are more similar to the human clinical phenotypes).

Rationale. Studies on animal models are critical for our understanding of the pathogenic mechanisms. More sophisticated animal models for FXTAS that more closely parallel the features seen in humans will facilitate the dissection of mechanism, thus revealing potential therapeutic targets. Furthermore, refined animal models provide the necessary foundation for testing of therapeutic agents prior to Phase I studies in humans.

Impact. Studies in appropriate animal models are essential for the development of candidate therapeutic agents that can then proceed to testing in human drug trials. Thus, such studies provide an incubator for the next generation of targeted treatments for FXTAS. Of much broader significance, however, is the potential of such studies — and the therapies developed through such studies — to reveal treatment approaches to other neurodegenerative disorders, such as Alzheimer and Parkinson diseases.

Goal 2 — Defining FXTAS Clinical Phenotypes

Recent studies suggest that FXTAS is a spectrum disorder that often involves, in addition to tremor and ataxia, a broad range of other neurological, as well as psychiatric and cognitive, problems that include nerve conduction abnormalities, autoimmune disease, anxiety and depression, and dementia. Research is needed to identify the full range of the clinical spectrum of FXTAS in order to discover pathogenic mechanisms and guide treatment. The risk and protective factors, and the prevalence of the disease within clinical groups, are largely unknown, making it very difficult to determine which individuals are at greatest risk for developing FXTAS. Prospective longitudinal studies, as well as studies of the natural course of FXTAS, are needed to better understand the rate of progression of the condition, whether an early prodromal state can be identified, and how to identify those at risk who may benefit from neuroprotective treatment. Understanding the natural history of FXTAS is crucial to being able to identify the impact of future treatment on the time course of disease. The formal process of validation of tools to quantify clinical involvement for various clinical domains (e.g., clinimetric analysis; inter-rater reliability) is crucial for characterization of disease features and relating these to molecular and other parameters, tracking the time course of disease progression, and monitoring potential effect of treatments.

The characterization of the full range of clinical effects of the fragile X premutation, its natural course, and the identification of the earliest markers of FXTAS disease are likely to lead to much more favorable outcomes and possibly to the prevention of disease in some individuals. The demonstration of therapeutic efficacy when monitoring treatment in clinical trials or general medical practice will depend on reliable, valid, and change-sensitive clinical instruments.

Objective 2.1. Define the broader range of neurological, neurocognitive, behavioral, and emotional dysfunction associated with FXTAS.

Rationale. Recent work suggests that aging individuals with the *FMR1* premutation may develop a much broader range of neurological, emotional, and cognitive symptoms than are described in the narrow currently accepted diagnostic criteria for FXTAS.

Impact. Definition of the full range of clinical effects of the *FMR1* premutation will facilitate diagnosis and proper management of problems in premutation carriers and, given the prevalence of the premutation, could potentially have a substantial impact on management and genetic counseling for a large number of individuals in the general population.

Objective 2.2. Develop and validate instruments that quantify clinical signs, including motor and neuropsychological signs, and progression of disease and instruments that are sensitive to early signs of FXTAS progression; identify the most sensitive and predictive parameters to include in these instruments through clinimetric testing.

Rationale. As neuroprotective and neurotherapeutic agents are developed, it will be essential to have a battery of well-validated and sensitive instruments to identify individuals at high-risk for or in the early stage of FXTAS and to enroll these individuals in clinical trials for outcomes measurement. Instruments should be sensitive enough to identify very early signs of disease.

Impact. Development of such instruments would result in improved, objective clinical characterization of premutation carriers with symptoms of FXTAS, the progress of their symptoms over time, and their response to therapeutic interventions.

Objective 2.3. Identify molecular, clinical, and environmental risk and protective factors associated with the penetrance of FXTAS.

Rationale. The fact that not all individuals who are carriers of premutation forms of the *FMR1* gene will develop FXTAS (incomplete penetrance) implies that factors other than the expanded repeat also play roles in the development of the disorder. This conclusion, in turn, implies that there are other genetic and/or environmental factors that confer additional risk or protection from disease occurrence and progression. Identification of these additional factors may provide new clues as to treatments or efforts to either reduce the severity of FXTAS or prevent its occurrence.

Impact. The identification of risk and protective factors may lead to interventions or lifestyle modifications in premutation carriers that reduce their risk for disease.

Objective 2.4. Prospectively identify the natural history of the *FMR1* premutation carrier and FXTAS progression, including factors associated with rapid and slow progression of disease.

Rationale. While it is evident from case reports that some affected persons have highly variable rates of disease progression, it is unknown what the usual rate of progression is and what factors slow or exacerbate progression.

Impact. This knowledge would improve the ability of individuals and families with FXTAS to cope with the disorder and plan for the future. Knowledge of factors that slow or exacerbate disease progression would shed light on the pathophysiology of the disease and may offer affected persons the potential to slow the disease's progression and/or offer unaffected carriers methods to reduce risk of disease.

Objective 2.5. Define the relationship between the FXTAS clinical phenotype, *FMR1* molecular genetic abnormalities, imaging, and measures of cellular pathology; identify factors (molecular, clinical, environmental) associated with various FXTAS clinical signs.

Rationale. Affected persons have a range of clinical signs, e.g., some have prominent dementia and little tremor while others have prominent tremor and minimal cognitive impairment. The molecular, cellular, and imaging abnormalities associated with various phenotypes are unknown. Further, the specific factors that predispose a person to have a specific clinical sign, e.g., frontal executive dysfunction, are unknown.

Impact. This knowledge would improve understanding of the pathophysiology of FXTAS. Moreover, the delineation of the relative impact of these various factors associated with the development of FXTAS signs may lead to a broader range of interventions to prevent or slow progression of disease.

Goal 3 — Epidemiology of FXTAS and *FMR1* Premutation Alleles

The incidence of FXTAS is currently unknown, and estimates are drawn from frequency measures for large normal and premutation repeat-length alleles in the general and in more restricted populations. However, the incomplete penetrance of FXTAS, coupled with the potential for poorly defined clinical phenotypes, suggests the need for more detailed surveys to establish the prevalence of FXTAS and related neurological disorders that result from *FMR1* premutation alleles.

Epidemiological data will determine the significance of FXTAS as a public health problem and help in developing strategies to approach individuals with FXTAS and their families for clinical studies.

Objective 3.1. Define the prevalence of the *FMR1* allele lengths in the general population ascertained in an unbiased fashion. Categorize these data for age; data across numerous age cohorts is desirable.

Rationale. Defining the frequency of expanded forms of the fragile X gene in the general population, and in an unbiased fashion, is critical for assessing the societal impact of FXTAS. At the present time, there is no unbiased estimate for premutation frequency in any large-scale population in the United States.

Impact. FXTAS may be among the most common single-gene causes of late-onset neurodegeneration in the United States. Unlike the majority of cases of late-onset Parkinson or Alzheimer disease, which are sporadic, the genetic basis of FXTAS allows estimates to be made for the total population at risk. As targeted therapies are developed, the ability to screen provides the added advantage of identification of individuals for preemptive therapeutic intervention.

Objective 3.2. Determine the prevalence of expanded *FMR1* alleles in adults with genetically undefined movement disorders (e.g., ataxia, tremor, Parkinsonism), memory impairment or dementia (e.g., Lewy body dementias, Alzheimer disease), dysautonomia, and/or peripheral neuropathy.

As a component of this Objective, additional consideration might be given as to how to establish the appropriate high-risk groups for screening. In particular, movement disorders or dementia clinics may not be the most appropriate venue for screening, as sampling bias can be introduced. For example, only a small minority of individuals with FXTAS might visit dementia clinics.

Rationale. FXTAS usually presents as a movement disorder, with other, more variable, associated neurological, medical, and neuropsychiatric impairments. However, the disorder may present with one of the associated features (e.g., dementia), thus escaping recognition, particularly in the absence of a recognized family history of fragile X-related disorders. It is thus expected that carriers of premutation alleles of the *FMR1* gene will be increased in individuals with various disorders (e.g., Parkinson disease, ataxia, dementia) that have substantial clinical overlap with FXTAS. Screening studies of these "high-risk" populations will identify the extent to which FXTAS cases are present within cohorts with a differing initial diagnosis.

Impact. Identification of appropriate high-risk populations would enhance the diagnostic opportunity for FXTAS.

Objective 3.3. Identify potential familial predisposition to FXTAS, its association with FXPOI and FXS, and find molecular factors involved in family clustering.

Rationale. Preliminary observations provide strong support for familial clustering of FXTAS cases within families, suggesting the presence of genetic or environmental factors common to these affected family members. In many cases, the study of families with a heavy burden of clinical involvement, or those with almost no involvement other than the initial diagnosis, provides the only means for identifying the second-gene effects. In the same vein, studies of such families may reveal different exposures (i.e., toxic chemicals, medications used to treat other disorders, etc.) that will lead to the identification of environmental influences.

Impact. Documenting the familial predisposition to FXTAS will provide the basis for sound clinical management of the entire family of the individual first identified with FXTAS. It will identify the familial relationships between neuroendocrine problems leading to POI and those leading to FXTAS, and it will help to identify the linkage between them. One of the major consequences of this understanding is cross-communication between clinical domains (obstetrics and gynecology, neurology, etc.).

Goal 4 — Early Diagnosis/Identification of Individuals Most At Risk of Developing FXTAS

Although the ascertainment of a CGG repeat in the premutation range confers carrier status and therefore the *a priori* possibility of developing FXTAS because longer repeats are associated with increased relative risk, neither the presence of a CGG repeat nor its length provides an accurate individual risk. There are carriers with a large premutation who never get disease and carriers with a small premutation who get relatively severe disease. In particular, it is very difficult to identify which female carriers are in the 8 percent to 10 percentwho are at increased risk for FXTAS, as this is dependent on both repeat length and activation ratios, and even these parameters together are poor predictors. This increased risk no doubt reflects underlying interacting genetic and environmental factors that have yet to be defined.

Studies in this area will lead to improved early diagnosis and knowledge of an individual's risk for FXTAS. This will enable clinicians to provide prognostic information that will help families with planning for the future, enable the identification of individuals most appropriate for studies of preventative treatments targeting the underlying mechanisms of cellular toxicity, and add to our knowledge of the complex interactions that predispose to FXTAS.

Objective 4.1. Develop molecular markers of cellular toxicity (e.g., metabolic, regulatory) that are assayable in a peripheral tissue or fluid of individual carriers to assist with prediction of impending disease before symptoms develop, finding those most at risk, and tracking cellular toxicity in carriers, with age, and after interventions.

Rationale. Whether an individual premutation carrier will develop FXTAS is unknown; this objective will provide metrics for involvement to be used for longitudinal studies.

Impact. This information will allow counseling of premutation carriers regarding their risk, will allow human studies to be focused on individuals at higher risk, and will allow tracking of the disease process at a cellular level.

Objective 4.2. Utilize these markers to assist with drug discovery for targeted treatments that block the mechanism of toxicity in the underlying disorder.

Rationale. No agents have been found that alter the pathophysiology of the disease; the development of markers will provide the necessary tools for assessing cellular response to candidate treatments for cellular toxicity.

Impact. Drugs that alter the disease process will be identified more efficiently, leading to clinical trials that are more likely to alter the course of the disease.

Objective 4.3. Develop radiological markers of CNS toxicity through more sensitive measures, such as DTI or MR spectroscopy (MR-SPECT), that will indicate individuals at risk for FXTAS before clinical symptoms or standard radiological signs of FXTAS become evident.

Rationale. Sensitive radiological markers have the potential to measure abnormal brain function representative of the disease process, thus identifying preclinical disease and individuals who may be at-risk for FXTAS.

Impact. This would allow *FMR1* premutation carriers to be counseled more accurately regarding their risk, and it will allow human studies to be focused on individuals at higher risk and allow tracking of the disease process radiologically.

Objective 4.4. Use the cellular, radiological, and clinical markers associated with FXTAS to successfully track improvements in toxicity measures with preventative or symptomatic treatment in clinical trials.

Rationale. No drugs have been shown to alter the pathophysiology of the disease or reduce symptoms; better quantifiers of CNS involvement are needed to measure CNS pathophysiology and therapeutic response.

Impact. This will allow confirmation of reversal of the disease process in human clinical trials of drugs or other agents.

Goal 5 — Supportive and Targeted Therapeutic Interventions for FXTAS

Currently there is no targeted treatment for FXTAS, and it is not known whether supportive treatments targeted to symptoms are truly helpful. Only one retrospective study exists to suggest that some individuals derive benefit from medication targeted to symptoms. Individuals with FXTAS are often treated with medications empirically, and these may be unhelpful or even detrimental; however, there is no information available to guide practice. Further, although there are likely to be some benefits of currently available supportive treatments, these are likely to be limited. Therefore, development of new therapeutics targeting the underlying disorder is crucial, and this can be aimed at both treatment to reduce symptoms and progression in symptomatic individuals and prevention of symptoms in at-risk presymptomatic individuals.

The identification of therapies that reduce symptoms will improve quality of life for those affected by FXTAS and potentially reduce burden on caregivers. Development of new therapies that slow or reverse the underlying disease or prevent FXTAS from occurring in those at risk would clearly provide a tremendous health-and-life benefit to fragile X premutation carriers and would reduce demands on public health resources.

Objective 5.1. Evaluate currently available pharmaceutical treatments targeted at specific symptoms in FXTAS to determine if they are helpful in well-designed clinical trials. Examples would be memantine for neurodegeneration and cognitive decline, minocycline and other putative neuroprotective agents, and standard treatments targeted at reduction of tremor.

Rationale. It is not currently known whether symptomatic medication treatments currently available are helpful, have no effect, or have deleterious effects in FXTAS.

Impact. Identification of helpful supportive medication therapies would improve quality of life and reduce burden for those with FXTAS and their families, while understanding which treatments provide no benefit or elicit negative effects would prevent fruitless treatment with such agents and exposure to unnecessary side effects.

Objective 5.2. Evaluate existing supportive devices and physical therapies to determine if these improve outcome (e.g., increase time to becoming wheelchair bound) or lengthen survival of persons with FXTAS.

Rationale. Persons with FXTAS have progressive loss of balance until they are confined to a wheelchair. Many have worsening action tremor that interferes with writing, eating, and other routine daily activities. Persons with FXTAS also become progressively weaker as they are forced to reduce activity due to their neurological symptoms. It is not currently known whether supportive devices and physical therapies can improve quality of life and adaptive skills in individuals with FXTAS. Many different types of canes and walkers and varied exercise programs are available, but use of these assistive walking devices and various exercise therapies in FXTAS has not been studied. Similarly, devices that reduce tremor are useful in other disorders but have not been studied in FXTAS. Of note, the provision of therapies that have no benefit is a waste of resources.

Impact. Identification of successful devices and physical therapies could improve quality of life, lengthen life span, and reduce burden for individuals with FXTAS and their families. The use of assistive walking devices and participation in exercise programs that reduce falls would reduce associated morbidity, e.g., hip and other fractures, head injuries. This would also increase the mobility of affected persons, increasing the likelihood that the individual with FXTAS and their family will interact more with others and improve the quality of their lives during their later years. Devices that compensate for tremor will improve the individual's ability to care for themselves and reduce caregiver burden. Furthermore, identification of non-beneficial supportive devices and physical therapies would prevent fruitless waste of resources.

Objective 5.3. Evaluate new drugs currently in development (e.g., oxybate, mGluR5 blockers) that are targeted to FXTAS symptoms in trials in animal models and human clinical trials.

Rationale. New drugs are being developed for common, well-known disorders, e.g., Parkinson disease and essential tremor, which have symptoms that also occur in FXTAS. For example, Parkinson disease and FXTAS have stiffness and cognitive dysfunction as common features, and both essential tremor and FXTAS have action tremor as a prominent symptom. Thus, drugs in development for Parkinson disease and essential tremor may reduce specific symptoms of FXTAS.

Impact. Identification of medications that control the symptoms of FXTAS would improve quality of life and reduce burden for those with FXTAS and their families. Drugs that reduce parkinsonian symptoms may reduce falls and the associated morbidity and would improve mobility. Drugs that reduce parkinsonian symptoms or tremor would allow the affected person to accomplish routine daily activities and reduce the need for caregiver assistance. Similarly, medications that benefit cognitive function would improve quality of life and reduce caregiver burden.

Objective 5.4. Utilize screening techniques that test the effect of large numbers of medications in cell culture and in animal models in reducing the toxic mechanisms that occur in FXTAS.

Rationale. Medications may currently be available that directly target the underlying mechanisms of cellular toxicity and may prevent, slow, or reverse the course of the disease itself but are not currently recognized as being of possible benefit for sufferers of FXTAS.

Impact. Discovery of such medications would lead to human clinical trials aimed at preventing, slowing, or reversing the underlying cellular toxicity that is the cause of FXTAS. Identification of these medications would result in reduced symptoms of FXTAS and longer life span. Reduced falls, tremor, and cognitive dysfunction would improve the quality of life of affected persons and their families because affected persons would have increased mobility, longer employment capability, and enhanced independence, mental health, and self care. Caregiver and family burden would be less, and ultimately there would be reduced demand on public health resources.

Objective 5.5. Evaluate novel therapeutic agents (e.g., RNAi, proteins or peptides, other small molecules) that may reverse cellular toxicity and may reverse or prevent FXTAS symptoms in animal models and in human clinical trials aimed at both treatment and prevention.

Rationale. Medications need to be developed that directly target the underlying mechanisms of cellular toxicity and prevent, reverse, or slow the disease itself but are not available for FXTAS.

Impact. Demonstration of the effectiveness of such medications would improve health and quality of life for persons with FXTAS, prevent or reduce suffering related to FXTAS, and reduce demands on public health resources to support individuals with FXTAS. Premutation carriers without FXTAS may also benefit greatly because such medications may spare them from developing the disorder or enable them to have a slower, less disabling progression of symptoms. Those with psychiatric symptoms may be less affected. Overall, quality of life would be improved for families with *FMR1* mutations.

Goal 6 — Quality-of-Life Issues Associated with FXTAS

Families with FXTAS struggle with many complex issues. Grandparents diagnosed with FXTAS feel guilt when they find that their grandchild's FXS is a result of a genetic mutation that the grandparent is carrying. The diagnosis of FXTAS in one individual of the family means all family members need to be counseled regarding their risks. The needs of the person with FXTAS drain the family's resources: financially, emotionally, and psychologically. The spouse of more than 40 years deals with an altered marital relationship as the affected person undergoes personality changes, develops dementia, and demands constant supervison. An elderly spouse has to figure out how and when to place her declining husband with FXTAS in a nursing home. Even though these challenging issues are common and obvious, there is little research to document the effects of FXTAS on quality of life, at the level of both the individual and the family. There is little information available on the impact of knowledge of premutation carrier status, and thus future risk of FXTAS, on quality of life. For example, how do individuals cope with the information that they are at risk for a neurodegenerative disorder? Is it best to be informed of one's premutation status in young adulthood and of one's risk for disease in later life, in light of the psychological stress that may occur over the years until symptoms begin, if they do at all? Data is also lacking regarding which symptoms of FXTAS are the most troublesome for the individual and their family. Further, the availability and adequacy of supportive services such as genetic counseling, family and individual counseling, and social work is unknown.

Understanding how the diagnosis of FXTAS or of the fragile X premutation carrier state affects quality of life will allow implementation of effective services to improve the quality of life of affected persons and their families. These services may include individual and marital counseling, programs to educate individuals with FXTAS and their families about the disorder, and provide adaptive guidance regarding changes in recreational and leisure activities and family structure. This would enhance opportunities to provide hope for affected families.

Objective 6.1. Assess the attitudes of individuals and their families about receiving a *FMR1* premutation diagnosis, the optimum time to receive this information, and their interest level regarding learning their carrier status to determine how much information may be shared with parents when a child is identified as being a carrier and who in the family needs to know.

Rationale. There is little consensus among researchers, clinicians, and families affected by FXS about the optimal time for individuals at risk for the premutation to be tested, or informed, and what kinds of information need to be conveyed, especially because the knowledge base regarding the FXTAS phenotype at different stages of development is rapidly expanding.

Impact. The information gained here will lead to more sensitive genetic counseling practices and better-defined recommendations for counseling individuals in FXTAS families.

Objective 6.2. Determine the availability and adequacy of genetic counseling for families, its usefulness and complexity, and the understandability of information provided through counseling after diagnosis as an *FMR1* premutation carrier.

Rationale. Knowledge regarding the genetics and phenotypes of fragile X-associated disorders is highly complex and can be confusing for families to understand. It is therefore imperative to develop readily available systems for the delivery of accurate information in a field that is rapidly changing.

Impact. Knowledge of the current status of effectiveness and accuracy of genetic counseling for *FMR1* mutations will lead to implementation of strategies that will reduce problems with omission of information and potentially damaging misinformation about the premutation carrier state and associated conditions.

Objective 6.3. Determine the impact of the *FMR1* premutation carrier diagnosis on the quality of life of the carrier individual and of other family members and design interventions to reduce negative effects on quality of life.

Rationale. Although clinical aspects of the *FMR1* carrier state are beginning to be elucidated, there is little, if any, information about how knowledge of carrier status affects the individual in his/her daily life or how family members are affected. Possible beneficial interventions include psychological counseling for the affected individual, family counseling, and genetic counseling.

Impact. This information will lead to practical, family-level interventions that may improve the quality of life for individuals who carry the *FMR1* premutation and their families.

Objective 6.4. Determine whether quality of life for those affected with FXTAS and their family members is most affected by motor, psychological/psychiatric, or cognitive dysfunction in the individual with FXTAS and determine which aspects of the quality of life are most affected.

Rationale. The broad spectrum of symptoms across neurological, cognitive, and psychiatric domains makes it difficult to determine the degree of impact of each of these problems in a person's daily life. Research aimed at identifying how certain symptoms relate to quality of life in areas such as interpersonal relationships, work, recreation, and self-care will lead to interventions that are more targeted and effective.

Impact. With this information, targeted interventions aimed at improving quality of life for individuals with FXTAS and their family members can be developed and, in conjunction with therapies reducing clinical symptoms, will lead to better outcomes for affected individuals and their families.

Objective 6.5. Develop, implement, and evaluate supportive interventions for individuals with FXTAS and their families.

Rationale. New supportive strategies are needed to help the many struggling families dealing with FXTAS. This disorder is novel and is distinct from other neurodegenerative disorders of the aging. For example, persons with Alzheimer disease have trouble finding words and tend to wander away but are not prone to falls, while individuals with FXTAS have minimal language difficulty but have poor insight and disinhibited behavior and fall easily. Research is needed that focuses on what supportive strategies (social, financial, emotional, medical) are most useful for individuals with FXTAS and their families.

Impact. Research that results in the availability of focused, beneficial services for individuals with FXTAS and their families will offer them needed support without wasting resources. For example, these strategies may improve the quality of psychological supportive services, genetic counseling, and counseling on financial and life planning. Availability of improved supportive interventions will improve quality of life for individuals with FXTAS and their families. For example, effective interventions aimed at increasing education about FXTAS may reduce anxiety and stress in individuals and family members, and counseling may help to improve marital and family relations that are affected by the development of degenerative disease in a loved one.

Objective 6.6. Determine the level of awareness among FXTAS-affected families regarding support systems at fragile X clinics and resource groups and their perception of need, adequacy, and availability of expertise in neurological management, psychological/counseling support, and availability of information on possible treatment options.

Rationale. It is unclear whether families with FXTAS are aware of support systems available to them, whether adequate resources for care exist, or whether families are availing themselves of these resources. It is important that resources are adequate and that affected persons are aware of them and thus able to use them.

Impact. Defining the availability and adequacy of currently available resources would prompt practitioners involved in these resources to improve their availability and the quality offered.

Goal 7 — Broader Implications for Other Neurodegenerative Diseases

The long-term objective of FXTAS research is to develop novel therapeutic strategies that will be broadly applicable to other late-onset neurodegenerative disorders, such as Parkinson and Alzheimer disease, where the specific causes of the late-onset forms of those diseases have not been identified. In this regard, the major advantage to other neurodegenerative disorders of studying FXTAS is that our knowledge of the triggering event (abnormal mRNA) in FXTAS will enable the study of the mechanisms of neural cell death that FXTAS has in common with other neurodegenerative disorders.

Detailed knowledge of the disease mechanism caused by *FMR1* premutation expansions in FXTAS will provide targets for treatments for FXTAS that are likely to be of much broader benefit to many forms of neurodegeneration involving movement disorders (e.g., Parkinson disease, Amyotrophic Lateral Sclerosis [ALS]) and dementias (e.g., Alzheimer disease, Parkinsonism with dementia).

Objective 7.1. Identify the disease pathways that are shared by FXTAS and more common neurodegenerative disorders, such as idiopathic Parkinson disease and Alzheimer disease.

Rationale. Common disease pathways are likely to be shared between FXTAS and more common neurodegenerative disorders. Identification of shared mechanisms will inform both FXTAS and other disorders in the areas of prevention and treatment. Common pathways provide the opportunity for common therapeutic interventions, and because the primary trigger for FXTAS is known, animal models can be established for studying the common pathways.

Impact. Development of targeted treatment strategies for a broad range of neurodegenerative disorders, based on studies of FXTAS, would have a huge social impact as treatments for the more common disorders are made available.

Objective 7.2. Determine the extent to which Parkinson disease-associated mechanisms (e.g., problems with the cell's ability to dispose of abnormally folded proteins, dysfunction of the energy-producing mitochondria, and oxidative damage) also play roles in FXTAS pathogenesis.

Rationale. Because FXTAS is associated with the formation of the same forms of particles ("inclusions") in the nuclei of neural cells as are found in other neurodegenerative disorders such as Huntington disease, similar pathogenic mechanisms are likely to be involved, such as the inability of the cell to dispose of abnormal protein aggregates or problems with energy generation in the cell.

Impact. To the extent that Parkinson disease-associated mechanisms are involved in FXTAS, which does have parkinsonism as a clinical feature, therapeutic approaches designed to target FXTAS will be applicable to Parkinson disease.

Objective 7.3. Determine whether the premutation influences the course of other neurodegenerative or non-CNS diseases.

Rationale. Additional neurodegenerative diseases (e.g., Huntington disease, myotonic dystrophy) are caused by microsatellite expansions, and there is now growing evidence that these disorders involve — at least in part — some of the same RNA-based causes of disease. Moreover, in Huntington disease as well as more than 100 other sites in the human genome, there are CGG-repeat elements that may also be associated with the disease process. Almost nothing is known about involvement of other CGG repeats.

Impact. Elucidation of the molecular etiology of FXTAS will likely also elucidate pathogenic pathways involved in other neurodegenerative disorders caused by unstable microsatellites, again offering up the prospect of common therapeutic approaches to more than a single disorder.

Infrastructure Needs
Objective 7.4. Develop conditional/inducible animal models that recapitulate specific neurotoxic events common to FXTAS and other neurodegenerative diseases.

Rationale. Conditional/inducible animal models have been used successfully to identify the sequence of pathogenic events in other inherited disorders, to understand the ability of tissues to recover after disease has begun, and to clarify the roles of specific disease factors. Animal models that can be induced to express a CGG-repeat element allow the study of the time course of events leading to disease.

Impact. Because our knowledge of the biochemical pathways involved in FXTAS disease progression is incomplete, these new models will provide critical information about the temporal and spatial development of CNS pathology. More specifically, identification of the earliest events following expression of the RNA will focus the targets for therapy.

Objective 7.5. Establish research initiatives and forums that promote collaborations between investigators studying FXTAS and other late-onset neurodegenerative disorders.

Rationale. Current programs fail to encourage effective interactions between investigators working on FXTAS and those working on other neurodegenerative disorders. New research strategies that promote such interactions will dramatically increase the rate of information transfer among laboratories with shared interest in neurodegenerative disorders, thus reducing the time involved with therapeutic development.

Impact. More effective communication between researchers working on different neurodegenerative diseases will promote a more rapid understanding of common mechanisms involved in neurodegeneration.

Goal 8 — Establishing a General Research Infrastructure for FXTAS

Sufficient general research infrastructure is critical to provide a foundation for research on the cause and disease mechanisms of FXTAS and for developing effective therapeutic interventions.

Establishing a general research infrastructure will be important for accomplishing all of the goals set forth for FXTAS research. Specifically, it will reduce the time involved in the development of targeted therapies for a variety of important neurodegenerative disorders through more efficient pooling of resources to define therapeutic targets that such disorders have in common.

Preclinical Research Infrastructure
Objective 8.1. Establish standardized endpoints for preclinical trials in animal models and ensure that facilities are available that enable testing of drugs and other therapeutic approaches.

Rationale. Standardized endpoints (e.g., improvement/remission from specific disease features) and established facilities for drug testing are important for preclinical trials across different institutions. When considering the efficacy of any new drug, particularly for neurodegenerative disorders whose clinical features are complex, clinical endpoints/successful outcomes should be carefully defined. For Parkinson disease, these would be reduction/elimination of tremor, reduction in stiffness, and improved cognitive abilities; for Alzheimer disease, such outcomes would include improved performance on memory tasks. Also, such endpoints are important in testing drugs, because such therapeutic interventions may affect one feature — tremor— without affecting another — memory.

Impact. These endpoints/facilities are critical for therapeutic development to establish optimal remission from clinical abnormalities and to create a broad spectrum of interventions (i.e., for both movement disorder and memory). For any disorder with a complex clinical picture, not just those involving neurodegeneration, precise outcome measures are therefore critical. Moreover, such measures are also better able to gauge subtle side effects that may accompany the beneficial effects of a new drug.

Objective 8.2. Create a mechanism to maintain animal (e.g., mouse) models of FXTAS at approved vendors in a live state that are available for easy and rapid importation into academic colonies.

Rationale. The ready availability of different animal models to the research community is critical for understanding the disease pathogenesis of FXTAS. When an investigator recognizes a need for additional animals, or animals that express certain features of a disease, the lead time can be reduced from many months in some cases (when such animals are transferred from laboratory to laboratory) to a matter of weeks for procurement, particularly if such animals are kept in certified repositories.

Impact. Easy access to the animal models would promote the research in FXTAS. In the absence of such animal models — for defining the disease process, for development of targeted therapeutics, and for initial drug treatment trials (which are required prior to FDA approval for use in human trials) — new drugs targeted to a specific disorder will not be developed.

Objective 8.3. Encourage the development of cell-based assays (e.g., stem cell-based technologies) that target aspects of pathogenesis and pathophysiology in FXTAS.

Rationale. To identify the effective compounds, the development of cell-based assays would be needed for high-throughput screens, that is, assays that are capable of processing thousands or millions of candidate drugs in a matter of weeks or months prior to any testing in whole animals. This approach not only saves years of work to refine the list of candidate drugs but also avoids the use of much larger animals for simple screening tasks.

Impact. The development of cell-based assays is critical for therapeutic development, because appropriate cell models, that is, cells that display features of the disease being studied, will save time, money, and the need for very large numbers of animals (e.g., mice) that would otherwise be needed for initial screening. Because we now know how to build adequate cell models for FXTAS, this disorder can serve as a paradigm for such studies.

Clinical Research and Trial Infrastructure
Objective 8.4. Establish a *FMR1* premutation patient registry and clinical data and sample repositories, including DNA, cells, and tissues.

Rationale. A patient registry of individuals with a *FMR1* premuation would be important for clinical research and clinical trials for associated disorders. Such a registry would allow the benefits and side effects of candidate drugs to be assessed in much larger populations. Such registries would also provide the foundation for the larger clinical trials that are necessary not only for evaluation of treatment strategies for the neurodegenerative disorders with complex clinical presentations such as FXTAS but also FXPOI.

Impact. Establishment of a good patient registry would have a huge impact on the success of therapeutic development and future clinical research because only through such registries, and the participation of the individuals participating in the registries, will optimal treatments be developed.

Objective 8.5. Develop a consortium of clinics to work with individuals with FXTAS, where there would be expertise in the use of optimal outcome measures and through which clinical trials could be run at multiple sites in a standardized fashion for future multicenter trials.

Rationale. Clinic consortia would facilitate the numbers of subjects required for detailed clinical trials and would in the interim help with the development of optimal outcome measures and diagnostic standards that are necessary for future multicenter trials.

Impact. Utilization of the clinic consortia will substantially reduce the time required to set up and evaluate multiple smaller trials for new drugs. Moreover, such smaller trials may lack sufficient statistical power to adequately evaluate targeted therapies for FXTAS and for related disorders.

Objective 8.6. Monitor, coordinate, and communicate the rehabilitation and educational assessment activities of the various federal agencies and voluntary and advocacy groups.

Rationale. The development of effective treatments for FXTAS will require close collaboration among federal agencies, researchers, and advocacy groups in order to adequately fund such large efforts and to facilitate the recruitment of large patient and control groups. Because such efforts are generally daunting for individual investigators, the proposed objective will facilitate this process.

Impact. Development of the lines of communication will promote research and therapeutic development for FXTAS as well as the transfer of information gained through FXTAS research to other neurodegenerative disorders.

Communication and Education

Objective 8.7. Design and implement a Web site that provides information and links to all existing FXTAS resources in both the United States and internationally.

Rationale. The Web site with the information on FXTAS will provide a forum for individuals with FXTAS to receive additional information and for researchers to recruit potential research participants to get involved in clinical research or clinical trials. Such a site will differ from current sites in being much more fully integrated across existing sites and groups, and it will be linked to sites that are more focused on other neurodegenerative disorders. Such multitiered linkage will foster the exchange of information across disorders in a manner that does not now occur.

Impact. It will increase the awareness of FXTAS and promote the interactions among individuals with FXTAS, clinical doctors, and basic researchers.

Objective 8.8. Stimulate international collaborations and infrastructure sharing to ensure that opportunities in FXTAS research are exploited and resources are used to maximum advantage.

Rationale. International collaboration will increase our understanding of FXTAS and promote therapeutic development for FXTAS.

Impact. Such collaborative efforts will help to define ethnic and geographical differences in the way the disease presents itself, thus defining additional factors that influence the disease process. Moreover, such collaborations foster stronger scientific/medical ties across cultures.

FXPOI SUMMARY OF GOALS AND OBJECTIVES

Estimated time to accomplish goal: short-term (ST), zero to three years; intermediate-term (IT), four to six years; long-term (LT), seven to ten years.
Perceived risk in terms of success: low risk (LR), moderate risk (MR), high risk (HR).

Goal I – Disease-Specific Mechanism and Therapeutic Targets

Develop model systems in which expanded FMR1 CGG repeats provoke the reproductive phenotype observed in humans in order to identify a mechanism and determine the time course of reproductive function (ST, MR).	Identify the reproductive, neuroendocrine, and other biological systems affected by the high CGG repeat (IT, LR).	Determine the specific molecular mechanism that causes the CGG repeat to be toxic to the reproductive, neuroendocrine, and other biological systems (IT, LR).	Investigate the association between FMR1 repeat size and reproductive phenotype in women to identify disease mechanism (IT, LR).	Identify targeted treatment strategies that extend the reproductive health of a FMR1 premutation carrier (LT, HR).	Identify common pathways of ovarian dysfunction between FXPOI and other forms of ovarian insufficiency (LT, LR).

Goal II – FXPOI Disease Progression and Preventive Medicine

Establish cross-sectional and longitudinal studies of hormonal, neuropsychological, and neuropsychiatric profiles, menstrual cycle alterations, fertility, and menopause transition in FMR1 premutation carriers (ST, LR).	Characterize menopausal symptoms, estrogen deficiency-associated disorders, androgen deficiency-associated disorders, neuropsychological and neuropsychiatric profile, and other reproductive-related disorders (e.g., cancers, endometriosis) and hypothalamic and pituitary function among FMR1 premutation carriers (ST, LR).	Identify biomarkers that predict reproductive health and establish a prospective study to determine their efficacy (IT, MR).

Goal III – Genetic and Environmental Factors that Influence Onset and Severity of FXPOI

Characterize effects of potential genetic and environmental modifying factors on qualitative and quantitative traits of FXPOI (ST, LR).	Conduct genetic and epigenetic studies among premutation carriers to identify genes and epigenetic factors that modify the onset and severity of reproductive phenotypes (LT, HR).

Goal IV – Diagnosis, Treatment, and Management of FXPOI

Establish best genetic counseling guidelines for FMR1 premutation carriers regarding the risk for fragile X-associated	Identify counseling strategies to facilitate effective family communication, enhance coping and adjustment to	Determine the best reproductive counseling and standard of care for an asymptomatic carrier of the FMR1 premutation, and	Estimate the frequency distribution of CGG repeats among women with ovarian insufficiency by ethnic group (ST,	Assess current treatments for infertility, menopause transition, osteoporosis, and other estrogen and	Determine the symptoms that may trigger a FMR1 diagnostic test among females of all ages. Generate public awarness	Determine the role of fertility preservation in females with FMR1 premutation who are deemed to have high risk of FXPOI	Establish clinical trials to examine efficacy of treatment strategies for reproductive health based on identified

disorders and for women with ovarian insufficiency regarding the risk for carrying the premutation; and develop education materials about fragile X-associated disorders (ST, LR).	fragile X-associated disorders (S-M-LT/MR).	determine the ethical, legal, and social issues of reproductive counseling for minors (IT, LR).	LR).	androgen deficiency-related health problems in *FMR1* premutation carriers based on existing clinical data (IT, LR).
				that early symptoms, such as altered menstrual cycles, are important to general health (ST, LR).
				(IT, MR).
				mechanism of *FMR1* repeat (LT, HR).

Goal V – Infrastructure Needs

Make FXPOI model systems available to researchers in order to identify mechanism and examine potential treatment time points to determine the time course of reproductive function (ST, LR).	Establish clinical fragile X research consortium to share knowledge, data, and biological samples (ST, LR).	Expand infrastructure to integrate knowledge from fragile X-associated disorders to increase cross-disciplinary studies (MR, LR).
		Develop education tools and methods to effectively disseminate knowledge to the public and to health professionals about fragile X-associated disorders (IT, LR).

61

FRAGILE X-ASSOCIATED PRIMARY OVARIAN INSUFFICIENCY (FXPOI)

GOAL 1 — FXPOI Disease-specific Mechanism and Therapeutic Targets

In contrast to FXS and FXTAS, little is known about the underlying pathophysiology and molecular mechanisms underlying FXPOI. While carriers of the full fragile X mutation do not transcribe the *FMR1* gene or produce the protein FMRP, premutation carriers produce *FMR1* transcripts with large CGG-repeat tracks (rCGGs). Furthermore, *FMR1* transcript levels increase with increasing repeat size, but levels of the protein FMRP are slightly decreased. Because FXTAS and FXPOI have been demonstrated only among premutation carriers, these disorders are unlikely to be the result of decreased protein. Rather, studies in animal models of FXTAS suggest that the large track of rCGGs acts in a toxic manner, perhaps by inactivating or sequestering other proteins.

Our understanding of the mechanism for FXPOI lags far behind the FXTAS field: there is no well-described model system for FXPOI, and to date, parallels to the FXTAS mechanism are untested hypotheses. The specific effects of the high CGG repeat on reproductive biology are unknown, but they need to be understood to effectively identify potential treatments.

Objective 1.1. Develop model systems in which expanded *FMR1* CGG repeats provoke the reproductive phenotype observed in humans in order to identify a mechanism and determine the time course of reproductive function.

Rationale. Human studies of FXPOI are limited to clinical descriptions and genetic and hormonal profiles. To thoroughly explore the disease mechanisms, we need animal models with varying number of CGG repeats, unstable repeats, and cell-type-specific inducible and conditional expression of the CGG repeats. Currently, two *fmr1* premutation mouse models exist that recapitulate the FXTAS phenotype, but their reproductive function has not been studied. Their characterization is urgently needed to know if these mice are useful models of human FXPOI. If not, other model systems need to be developed to understand the pathophysiology and molecular consequences of the high CGG repeat.

Impact. Model systems have proven invaluable for studies of both FXS and FXTAS. Once FXPOI pathophysiology is understood in animal models, translational studies can begin to identify prognostic and treatment strategies for women with the premutation.

Objective 1.2. Identify the reproductive, neuroendocrine, and other biological systems affected by the high CGG repeat.

Rationale. At least some women with the fragile X premutation and regular menstrual cycles have signs of early ovarian aging and follicle loss (elevated FSH and decreased inhibin B levels and lower anti-mullerian hormone [AMH] levels) compared to noncarriers. However, it is unclear which system is affected by the CGG repeat to cause early ovarian aging. For example, the effect of the repeat could target a specific stage of follicle development. Alternatively, it could cause alterations in the hypothalamic-pituitary-gonadal (HPG) axis.

Impact. It is imperative to understand the biological system that is influenced by high CGG repeats in order to determine prognostic and treatment strategies. These studies, done in parallel with those in model systems, will identify the target(s) of the toxic effect of the high repeat and provide strategies to ameliorate ovarian insufficiency.

Objective 1.3. Determine the specific molecular mechanism that causes the CGG repeat to be toxic to the reproductive, neuroendocrine, and other biological systems.

Rationale. With the precedents of FXTAS and other repeat-sequence disorders, changes in *FMR1* RNA are hypothesized to cause reproductive dysfunction in women with the *FMR1* premutation. The RNA effects might be related to increased *FMR1* mRNA levels or its unusual structure due to the large repeat tracks. This structure could inactivate other proteins by binding them, targeting them for degradation, or sequestering them. It is also possible that the repetitive elements in the premutation *FMR1* transcript act through RNA interference to silence genes with short complementary repeats in their transcripts. FXTAS cells have intranuclear inclusions that, while not pathogenic, stain with anti-ubiquitin antibodies, suggesting a link to proteasome protein degradation. These as well as other possible mechanisms need to be tested to understand the disease process in FXPOI.

Impact. Understanding the molecular consequence of high CGG repeats will determine which properties can be altered by therapeutic agents to reduce toxic effects. This strategy has been exploited very successfully in studies of FXS and FXTAS.

Objective 1.4. Investigate the association between *FMR1* repeat size and reproductive phenotype in women to identify disease mechanism.

Rationale. It is important to note that the *FMR1* repeat classification system of "premutation" and "noncarrier" relates only to the risk for instability and expansion to the full mutation; they do not necessarily correspond to the risk for premutation-associated disorders such as FXPOI. Studies to identify at-risk alleles have not been completed.

The degree of ovarian dysfunction in women with the *FMR1* premutation depends on repeat size, but the relationship is not linear: women with mid-range repeats (80 to 100 repeats) have earlier and more severe ovarian dysfunction than women with smaller or larger premutations. It is possible that the mid-range repeat lengths result in the greatest amount of mRNA and therefore the greatest toxicity or that the mid-range repeat confers a specific mRNA conformation that interacts with different proteins or mRNAs.

Impact. Understanding the molecular consequence of high CGG repeats will determine which properties can be altered by therapeutic agents to reduce toxic effects. Furthermore, it is important to determine the characteristics of the structure of the repeat (size and AGG interspersion pattern) that increase risk for reproductive dysfunction, to better counsel asymptomatic women with the premutation.

Objective 1.5. Identify targeted treatment strategies that extend the reproductive health of a *FMR1* premutation carrier.

Rationale. No treatment strategy based on the underlying mechanism of the CGG repeat has been identified to extend the reproductive health of a carrier with the premutation. At this time, the symptoms are treated based on current knowledge of other forms of ovarian insufficiency, but their effectiveness is variable or unknown at this time.

Impact. Treatment regimes based on the underlying molecular mechanisms and identified biological systems affected by the *FMR1* CGG repeat will be the most effective. Importantly, it may be possible to treat women who carry high-risk *FMR1* alleles *prior to the onset of obvious reproductive dysfunction*, as carriers can be identified easily by molecular tests at any point in their lifetime.

Objective 1.6. Identify common pathways of ovarian dysfunction between FXPOI and other forms of ovarian insufficiency.

Rationale. Understanding the pathways involved in FXPOI may shed light on the study of other systems that might be perturbed in other forms of ovarian insufficiency. These can be efficiently investigated using the tools developed for FXPOI. In addition, the effect of the *FMR1* CGG repeat size on ovarian function may be modified by other genes that lead to POI, either interacting in the same pathway or adding to their effect.

Impact. The cause of more than 80 percent of POI is unknown. *FMR1* premutation is one of the few known causes, and women at risk can be identified prior to the onset of symptoms. Knowledge of the mechanism underlying FXPOI could help us identify other causes of POI and increase the reproductive health of many individuals. Investigating the impact of other known genes for POI on ovarian function in women with the premutation and a variable number of CGG repeats will unravel the variability in ovarian function in women who have a similar number of CGG repeats.

GOAL 2 — FXPOI Disease Progression and Preventive Medicine

POI cannot be predicted in a majority of cases, nor can the longitudinal course of ovarian function be predicted. Because *FMR1* premutation status can be determined before the onset of any pathology, longitudinal studies of fragile X premutation carriers would grant us a unique opportunity to examine the course of FXPOI, from elevated FSH levels with regular menses to irregular or missed menstrual cycles, infertility, menopause before the age of 40 years, or early menopause (compared to controls). Associated symptoms, including estrogen deficiency and its consequent osteoporosis and cardiovascular risk, can also be defined.

Studies in human *FMR1* premutation carriers and mouse models raise the possibility that other endocrine and neuroendocrine organs are affected. Intranuclear inclusions have been found in the pituitary and adrenal glands and in the testicular Leydig cells of *FMR1* premutation carriers.

Thus, additional studies are needed to define reproductive and endocrine manifestations in the pituitary, gonads, and adrenal glands of both men and women.

The relationship of the endocrine disorders to the neuropsychiatric manifestations also needs investigation. Men and women with FXTAS symptoms reported higher levels of several types of psychological symptoms compared to published norms, possibly due to adrenal gland dysfunction. There also appears to be an increased risk for the development of mood disorders in some women during the menopausal transition.

Identifying women who carry the fragile X premutation provides a unique opportunity to identify women at risk for POI and to study the biomarkers that might predict the longitudinal course of the disease. Identifying these biomarkers will also be critical to counsel individual women about their reproductive potential.

Objective 2.1. Establish cross-sectional and longitudinal studies of hormonal, neuropsychological, and neuropsychiatric profiles, menstrual cycle alterations, fertility, and menopause transition in *FMR1* premutation carriers.

The short-term goal is to establish longitudinal studies to examine the course of ovarian function in fragile X premutation carriers. These studies will require a collaborative network and definition of the parameters for measurement, such as the history, physical exam, and serum biomarkers. The intermediate goal is to define the course of reproductive function using data obtained from a longitudinal study of fragile X premutation carriers.

Rationale. See overall rationale for Goal 2.

Impact. Determining the time course of the reproductive abnormalities associated with premutations could have an enormous impact on counseling about prognosis, fertility potential, fertility risks such as IDD, and fertility treatment. From a broader health perspective, the time course could also impact counseling regarding the risks for osteoporosis and cardiovascular disease.

Objective 2.2. Characterize menopausal symptoms, estrogen deficiency-associated disorders, androgen deficiency-associated disorders, neuropsychological and neuropsychiatric profile, and other reproductive-related disorders (e.g., cancers, endometriosis) and hypothalamic and pituitary function among *FMR1* premutation carriers.

Rationale. See overall rationale for Goal 2.

Impact. Defining these characteristics will help develop recommendations for testing for estrogen deficiency-associated disorders, alert physicians to possible need for counseling or psychiatric referral, and help women consider possible treatment options for menopausal or neuropsychiatric symptoms. These studies will also determine whether men who carry the premutation need endocrine follow-up and whether follow-up needs to cover all of the neuroendocrine axes.

Objective 2.3. Identify biomarkers that predict reproductive health and establish a prospective study to determine their efficacy (also see Goal 3.1 in the following section).

The intermediate goal is to identify biomarkers of reproductive health, and the long-term goal is to use them to create a predictive model of reproductive function in fragile X premutation carriers and design a prospective study to establish their validity.

Rationale. Biomarkers that reflect reproductive function and capacity would be useful to predict reproductive function and the time to menopause in women who carry the fragile X premutation. Candidate biomarkers include follicle count and levels of the hormones FSH, inhibin A, inhibin B, and anti-mullerian hormone. AMH may be particularly important, as it appears to change ahead of other markers.

Impact. Determining the biomarkers that predict reproductive abnormalities associated with premutations could have an enormous impact on counseling about prognosis, fertility potential, fertility risks such as FXS, and fertility treatment, and could help define recommendations for testing. From a broader health perspective, the time course could also impact counseling regarding the risks of osteoporosis and cardiovascular disease. These studies will provide information that is critically important for the clinical care of women who carry the premutation and possibly a broader group of infertility patients.

GOAL 3 — Genetic and Environmental Factors that Influence Onset and Severity of FXPOI

Genetic markers (such as CGG repeat number, interspersed AGG sequences and X chromosome inactivation ratio [XCI]) and environmental factors (such as smoking) might also affect the reproductive life span in women and the hormonal profile of men and women who carry the *FMR1* premutation.

It is well documented that the *FMR1* alleles vary not only in CGG repeat number but also in patterns of AGG interspersion within the repeat tract. AGG interruptions decrease the risk for expansion of a premutation to a full mutation, and *in vitro*, they prevent the formation of branched hairpin structures, suggesting that AGG interspersions might alter the association between repeat size and presence of disease. In one small preliminary study, AGG interruption was correlated with a protective effect on ovarian aging. Thus, further examination is needed to determine the effects of interspersed AGG repeats, and other factors, on FXPOI.

Objective 3.1. Characterize effects of potential genetic and environmental modifying factors on qualitative and quantitative traits of FXPOI.

Rationale. Additional studies that examine potential *FMR1*-related risk factors in known premutation carriers are needed to provide prognostic indicators of the severity of the disorder. Both cross-sectional and cohort study designs would be useful and would be aided by large consortia. DNA samples and reproductive outcome measures such as age at menopause, number of live births, age at each live birth, number of miscarriages, and other reproductive information may be highly informative. Such data may be examined for the effects of presumed modifying factors (CGG repeat length, AGG interspersion, XCI, smoking) and other, currently unknown, risk factors on both qualitative traits (e.g., FXPOI) and quantitative traits (age at menopause, hormone levels, menstrual cycle characteristics, number of pregnancies, etc).

Impact. Determination of the relationship of modifying factors to FXPOI risk in a very large sample of women would provide insight into the biological mechanism of the CGG repeat. In addition, these data would provide predictive markers to increase the accuracy of counseling women who carry a premutation concerning their risk of FXPOI. It is possible that these data could also provide guidance for physicians treating such women. It is also possible that these data will help identify appropriate patients for clinical trials as treatments are developed.

Objective 3.2. Conduct genetic and epigenetic studies among premutation carriers to identify genes and epigenetic factors that modify the onset and severity of reproductive phenotypes.

Rationale. Results from family studies indicate that the age of menopause has a strong family component, even after the effect of CGG repeat size is removed. This suggests that there are other sources of genetic variation that contribute to the onset and severity of FXPOI.

Impact. Significant linkage and/or association of modifier loci for FXPOI would identify biological pathways that affect the penetrance of the premutation alleles. A better understanding of biological causation can lead to better methods for prevention and treatment of ovarian dysfunction in premutation carriers. In addition, identification of risk alleles would provide predictive information about ovarian dysfunction among women who carry the premutation. Such information would improve genetic counseling and provide better guidance for physicians.

GOAL 4 — Diagnosis, Treatment, and Management of FXPOI

Objective 4.1. Establish best genetic counseling guidelines for *FMR1* premutation carriers regarding the risk for fragile X-associated disorders and for women with ovarian insufficiency regarding the risk for carrying the premutation; and develop education materials about fragile X-associated disorders.

Rationale. Because fragile X-associated disorders are the result of an heritable, expanding triplet repeat mutation, the diagnosis of one individual has significant implications not only for their immediate family but also for extended relatives in multiple generations. Research is needed to develop strategies for families to help positively manage the information and to evaluate the effectiveness of these strategies. Outcomes-based research is critically needed to explore perceptions and understanding of genetic risk information, effect on the family, and adjustment to the variable implications of this disorder.

Most women with ovarian insufficiency express interest in carrier testing for fragile X, but women who are found to be premutation carriers are unprepared for their result. This indicates a strong need for genetic counseling for women at risk for FXPOI.

Women who need counseling for FXPOI could come from a family with FXS, or they could have no family history of FXS but experience ovarian insufficiency. Current protocols state that women who are *FMR1* premutation carriers should be informed about their risk for FXPOI, but there are limited guidelines for their genetic counseling. There are no guidelines regarding genetic counseling for women with ovarian insufficiency who are offered *FMR1* carrier testing through their specialist or for women identified as premutation carriers as a result of their ovarian insufficiency. Both groups of women need counseling as to reproductive options in view of a potentially reduced reproductive time span, the risk of having a child with FXS, and the health effects of potential early ovarian aging. Women without a family history of FXS need to learn about FXS and cope with the discovery of an inherited condition that might affect other family members.

Impact. Findings from this research will inform the development of best-practice guidelines, which will in turn improve the care of women with POI or who are at risk of FXPOI as a result of their premutation carrier status. Because FXPOI could be diagnosed before the onset of any symptoms, developing educational materials is essential in increasing awareness of FXPOI and fragile X-associated disorders among the general public and health care providers.

Objective 4.2. Identify counseling strategies to facilitate effective family communication, enhance coping and adjustment to fragile X-associated disorders.

(Note: We have included fragile X-associated disorders as well as FXPOI in this objective because women who have FXPOI will have relatives with fragile X-associatated disorders, and their experiences will impact on their coping, adjustment, and family communication.)

Rationale. The emotional strain of being identified as an *FMR1* premutation carrier goes beyond the individual because carriers then feel obligated to deliver this genetic and medical information to family members. At this time, there are few tools to help individuals do so, especially for the fragile X-associated disorders, where the inheritance of the mutation is complex and the association with different syndromes is unwieldy.

Impact. Research to guide the development of genetic counseling strategies will improve the care of women and their families. Informational materials will help educate women and health careproviders about all aspects of fragile X-associated disorders. Importantly, materials and strategies to help communicate information about fragile X-associated disorders to families are essential to all carriers of the *FMR1* mutation in any of its forms.

Objective 4.3. Determine the best reproductive counseling and standard of care for an asymptomatic carrier of the *FMR1* premutation, and determine the ethical, legal, and social issues of reproductive counseling for minors.

Rationale. FMR1 premutations are challenging to explain to patients and their families because of the complex inheritance involving repeat expansion and the different phenotypes that can be expressed. In addition to concerns women may have regarding the risk of having an affected child, they may feel pressured to have children earlier because of a potentially reduced reproductive time span, and they may suffer anxiety, guilt, and feelings of low self-worth. These issues become more complicated when an adolescent girl is diagnosed as an *FMR1* premutation carrier.

Impact. Identification of fragile X mutation carrier status allows girls and women to make informed reproductive decisions. A better understanding of the psychological impact of this condition, which affects future fertility in a girl or young woman,and how this relates to genetic counseling will permit the delivery of higher-quality, more sensitive interactions. This will improve long-term emotional health and permit individuals who carry the *FMR1* premutation to make reproductive choices that benefit their family and society.

Objective 4.4. Estimate the frequency distribution of CGG repeats among women with ovarian insufficiency by ethnic group.

Rationale. The prevalence of the fragile X premutation in women with early stages of POI is unknown. Approximately 20 percentof couples presenting for fertility treatment have evidence of these early stages of POI. These women might have a high risk of carrying a fragile X premutation and bearing a child with FXS.

Preliminary small reports suggest that women with ovarian dysfunction ranging in severity from early POI to end-stage POI (POF) have *FMR1* genes enriched for repeat lengths at the upper limit of normal (35 to 41 repeats) and in the intermediate range (55 to 58 repeats) compared to the general population. These findings point to the possibility that the repeat number in the *FMR1* gene may be related to ovarian function and dysfunction even within the normal range. These women are not at risk for bearing a child with FXS in one generation (Nolin et al., 2003). However, it is critical to determine the risk of FXPOI conferred by increasing CGG repeat number in the *FMR1* gene in a large cohort.

The frequency of the *FMR1* CGG repeat number differs among ethnic groups. Several large, population-based studies demonstrate that the prevalence ranges from 1/246 to 1/468 in Caucasian populations. In addition, it appears that there is variability at the fragile X locus that is dependent on ethnic background. For example, studies of the common repeat number and/or prevalence of the premutation have demonstrated a higher prevalence of the premutation in Israel, a similar prevalence of the repeat distribution and premutation in Caucasians and African Americans in the United States, but a smaller common repeat number in Chinese subjects. Thus, studies of *FMR1* premutation prevalence and distribution of the CGG repeat number in various ethnic populations in the United States will be necessary to determine the prevalence of the premutation, particularly among Asian Americans and other ethnic subgroups. In turn, the risk of ovarian dysfunction in these populations in relation to the distribution of the premutation needs definition.

Impact. Studying the prevalence of the fragile X premutation in women across the spectrum of POI and across ethnic groups along with the distribution of CGG repeats in women with POI is critical to determine the patient population requiring testing for the premutation. These studies may also point to the importance of determining the repeat number and define the repeat number that confers risk for FXPOI. These studies will be particularly important for women in their childbearing years, especially in the setting of infertility treatment. These studies will facilitate early detection of women at risk for infertility and the complications of estrogen deficiency. They also have the potential to prevent FXS. Finally, if there is a relationship between the CGG repeat number and FXPOI, these studies may identify one of the most important predictors of ovarian aging.

Objective 4.5. Assess current treatments for infertility, menopause transition, osteoporosis, and other estrogen and androgen deficiency-related health problems in *FMR1* premutation carriers based on existing clinical data.

Rationale. Currently, women who carry the *FMR1* premutation receive standard treatment for infertility, FXPOI, and early menopause, but its efficacy in these women is not known. These assessments can be made from existing clinical data or within clinical trials.

Impact. Studying the efficacy of infertility treatments and treatment designed to alleviate estrogen and androgen-deficiency complications will provide direct evidence for treatment recommendations in women who carry the fragile X premutation. In addition, if the women can be identified before the onset of problems, the infertility and sex hormone deficiency-related problems may be prevented. Therefore, these studies will be a catalyst to prospective disease prevention trials. Finally, these studies in women with FXPOI may be applicable to any woman who suffers from POI or to men and women who suffer from physiologic sex hormone deficiency in the perimenopause or andropause.

Objective 4.6. Determine the symptoms that may trigger a *FMR1* diagnostic test among females of all ages. Generate public awareness that early symptoms, such as altered menstrual cycles, are important to general health.

Rationale. It is imperative to define the clinical phenotype of ovarian insufficiency along the entire course of its development. Thus, assessment of the leading-edge symptoms among premutation carriers throughout all life stages is necessary to identify symptoms that may prompt *FMR1* testing among adolescents and women. This would permit earlier diagnosis. It is likely that for some young girls the leading-edge symptom will be failure of pubertal development, for some it may be the failure to establish regular ovulatory menstrual cycles, and for some the leading edge may be onset of secondary oligomenorrhea/amenorrhea or unexplained infertility.

Public awareness is key to help increase the number of early diagnoses. Evidence suggests that many women and clinicians do not take disturbances of the menstrual cycle seriously as a marker of a health disorder in need of evaluation. Women with primary ovarian insufficiency on average have to see three different health care providers before the diagnosis is confirmed by a simple blood test, and the median delay in diagnosis is two years.

Impact. Clear data regarding leading-edge symptoms will help clinicians use a more targeted approach when performing evaluations related to *FMR1* mutations. Early diagnoses can help prevent major health problems such as loss of bone density related to estrogen deficiency and will maximize the available reproductive options. Raised awareness will also generate more research and more training of clinicians interested in specializing in these disorders. This benefits many women by giving them more options and better health care overall.

Objective 4.7. Determine the role of fertility preservation in females with *FMR1* premutation who are deemed to have high risk of FXPOI.

Rationale. FXPOI is likely to be one of the very few conditions where risk of ovarian insufficiency can be judged prospectively. It also is likely to be one of the most common genetic conditions associated with future infertility: at least 20 percent of infertility patients have diminished ovarian reserve, and a significant proportion of these patients might carry the *FMR1* premutation or high-normal CGG counts.

Fertility preservation utilizes oocyte, embryo, and ovarian tissue cryopreservation as a safeguard against future infertility. There are no data available on how women with high CGG counts respond to ovarian stimulation regimens and how successful the cryopreservation technologies will be given the existing ovarian dysfunction. Timing of fertility preservation procedures as well as the ethical issues surrounding fertility preservation in children with high CGG repeats also needs to be studied.

Impact. FMR1 premutations may prove to be one of the most important determinants of future fertility and gonadal function. If appropriate fertility preservation techniques are determined for premutation carriers, preservation of gonadal function and fertility will have a significant and measurable impact on quality of life. For example, preservation and restoration of gonadal function by cryopreservation and future transplantation may prevent not only infertility but also menopause-related health issues.

Objective 4.8. Establish clinical trials to examine efficacy of treatment strategies for reproductive health based on identified mechanism of *FMR1* repeat.

Rationale. The overarching goal of research on FXPOI is to ameliorate the symptoms associated with FXPOI and extend the reproductive health of a premutation carrier. Once the mechanism of the toxic effect of the CGG repeat is established and potential treatment strategies are identified, clinical trials will be necessary. Thus, this aim can be accomplished with the culmination of the scientific endeavors outlined above and infrastructure outlined below.

Impact. Clinical trials are essential to determine efficacy of treatment. Information from these trials will determine the potential to treat infertility and treat estrogen and androgen-deficiency complications. In addition, trials to study treatments that are implemented prior to the onset of problems may prevent infertility and sex hormone deficiencies. Finally, these studies may be applicable to any woman who suffers from POI or men and women who suffer from physiologic sex hormone deficiency in the perimenopause or andropause.

GOAL 5 — Infrastructure Needs

As with FXS, most research to date in the area of FXPOI has relied on individual investigator-initiated efforts, with little in the way of broad infrastructure support. While this was sufficient in the early stages of research, the FXPOI field has made sufficient advances so that specific core supports would now enhance the quality, timeliness, and efficiency of research. Three examples of areas of needed infrastructure are: (1) a broader array of appropriate nonhuman models of fragile X-associated disorders easily accessible by researchers from a variety of institutions; (2) a human brain, gonad, and tissue bank; and (3) a patient registry or research consortium to maximize access to a large number of individuals with fragile X-associated disorders for both descriptive and intervention studies. Importantly, all of the information that comes from the essential research needs to be disseminated in a coordinated way to increase the translation to the health professionals and community.

Objective 5.1. Make FXPOI model systems available to researchers in order to identify mechanism and examine potential treatment time points to determine the time course of reproductive function.

Rationale. As mentioned in Goal 1, development of model systems for FXPOI is far behind FXS and FXTAS. The importance of the development of models is outlined above. Here we focus on ensuring that models are freely available to all researchers to enable progress to be made quickly and efficiently.

Impact. Remarkable progress can be made using shared resources and communicating results as quickly as possible. Development of model systems is expensive and labor-intensive. Once the system is established, work can proceed among many interested groups using various approaches.

Objective 5.2. Establish clinical *fragile X* research consortium to share knowledge, data, and biological samples.

Rationale. A large population of individuals is needed to understand the variable phenotype of those with *FMR1* mutations and to conduct studies to assess the safety and efficacy of interventions. The establishment of a tissue/blood/DNA bank would allow access to a large number of samples from individuals with *FMR1* mutations that could lead to research breakthroughs such as the discovery of biomarkers to predict ovarian function in premutation carriers. A large population in which to study the natural history of disease and interventions would have the statistical power to detect small, but clinically important, differences not detectable in smaller populations.

Clinics that specialize in treating and managing health care for patients with FXS and other fragile X-associated disorders provide a basis for a clinical research consortium. However, other clinic resources are needed to evaluate the natural history of disease and potential interventions in premutation carriers who may not have a family history of FXS, such as individuals diagnosed with FXPOI and FXTAS in fertility and neurology clinics. This population is important to

72

include in studies to evaluate differences between premutation carriers with or without a family history of FXS.

Collaboration between clinics is essential, as clinics that care for individuals and families with fragile X-associated disorders individually see small numbers of patients. Exisiting successful clinical consortia such as the Pediatric Oncology Group can be used as models for development of a consortium for fragile X research.

Impact. Establishment of a fragile x clinical consortium, and thus a large population of individuals with *FMR1* mutations, would increase our knowledge of fragile X-associated disorders (phenotype, prevalence, biomarkers, age of onset, associated modifying factors, etc.). Adding specialty clinics to the consortium would enable discovery of genetic and/or phenotypic differences between carriers identified through family history of FXS and those without such history. Researchers would be able to identify a large number of individuals eligible for clinical trials.

Objective 5.3. Expand infrastructure to integrate knowledge from fragile X-associated disorders to increase cross-disciplinary studies.

Rationale. Creating an infrastructure to integrate knowledge from all fragile X-associated disorders is essential to cross-fertilize the research on each disorder. It is clear that the *FMR1* premutation is toxic to the brain and gonadal tissues. The focus on only one target reduces the ability to treat the person as a whole.

Impact. Consolidating knowledge identified through the study of those with fragile X-associated disorders will help researchers, health care and educational professionals, and the community at large. It will advance the field rapidly and help coordinate findings relative to all *FMR1* mutation carriers.

Objective 5.4. Develop education tools and methods to effectively disseminate knowledge to the public and to health professionals about fragile X-associated disorders.

Rationale. Research findings need to be disseminated to facilitate the translation of findings into the clinical setting. Disseminating the latest research findings and educating health care providers and the public will increase knowledge and raise awareness about fragile X-associated disorders. Various forms of media will be required to reach these audiences. A significant body of research supports health education as a successful approach to improving knowledge, which in turn contributes to adopting health behaviors and utilization of resources to improve quality of life and health outcomes.

Impact. The impact of disseminating research findings will be to increase awareness of fragile X-associated disorders among health care providers and the general public. Translation of findings from the research to the clinical setting could improve diagnostic practices of physicians in identifying individuals with fragile X-associated disorders and improve treatment/outcomes for affected individuals.

SUMMARY OF SIMILARITIES AND DIFFERENCES IN RESEARCH PRIORITIES BETWEEN FXS AND ASSOCIATED DISORDERS

Differences and similarities in research needs between disorders were discussed by the three working groups jointly during the May 2008 Research Plan development meeting. This section identifies areas of overlap that were deliberated and is not considered to be exhaustive. For cross-referencing purposes, the goals identified by the working groups with the most significant commonalities identified are highlighted below.

FXS, FXTAS, and FXPOI all stem from mutations in the same part of the *FMR1* gene, and common research priorities are evident within the goals and objectives described in previous sections. While some of the goals for the three disorders appear to be the same, it must be noted that some of the objectives are actually dissimilar. There are several reasons for this. First and foremost, these disorders are completely different in whom they affect, age ranges of onset, and presumably mechanism of disease. Second, research on each disorder is at different levels of maturity, with FXS studied for decades and FXTAS and FXPOI only being recently indentified. For example, all three working groups emphasized the need for further research on disease mechanisms (pathophysiology) underlying the effects of *FMR1* mutations, but the research objectives for each disorder reflect differences in when, how, and in whom these mechanisms manifest in symptoms of FXS, FXTAS, or FXPOI.

Examples of research priorities with similar themes yet differing objectives by disorder:
1. Pathophysiology underlying consequences of FMR1 gene mutations, e.g., FXS (1.1–1.8), FXTAS (1.1–1.7), FXPOI (1.1–1.6).

2. Improving diagnosis, e.g., FXS (2.1–2.4), FXTAS (4.1–4.4), FXPOI (4.6–4.8).

3. Developing and assessing treatments and interventions, e.g., FXS (4.1–4.5), FXTAS (5.1–5.5), FXPOI (4.5).

While recognizing the distinctions between disorders is important it must be noted that there are also goals where the objectives overlap across the three disorders. For example, FXS, FXTAS, and FXPOI are heritable, and a single family may be impacted by not only one but possibly by all three disorders in both current and future generations. Thus, all three disorders may share similar needs and issues, particularly when addressing needs associated with family and when issues of testing and counseling and access to care are involved.

Examples of research priorities where goals overlap and opportunities for resource sharing and collaboration across disorders are possible:
4. Determining the population prevalence and incidence of FMR1 allele variants, e.g., FXS (2.3), FXTAS (3.1–3.3), FXPOI (4.4).

5. Impact on the family, e.g., FXS (5.1–5.3), FXTAS (6.1– 6.6), FXPOI (4.1–4.3).

6. Infrastructure to facilitate collaboration and data and resource sharing (e.g., tissue banking, education, registry), e.g., FXS (6.1–6.3), FXTAS (8.3–8.5), FXPOI (5.1–5.4).

RESEARCH PLAN IMPLEMENTATION

The *NIH Research Plan on Fragile X Syndrome and Associated Disorders* was developed with significant input from leading researchers and clinicians in each field along with families and advocate groups, representatives from the NIH FXRCG, parents, and participants from other federal agencies working collaboratively on the FXS, FXTAS, and FXPOI working groups. The goals and objectives for each disorder are intended to be comprehensive but by no means exhaustive and include research priorities that extend from "bench-to-bedside-to-community." Historically, NIH has taken the lead in basic science discoveries that will help drive treatment development and disease prevention, but some aspects of this Research Plan will be more appropriately addressed by other agencies or organizations. While the Research Plan is primarily intended to provide the ICs of NIH with guidelines for prioritizing future research related to FXS, FXTAS, and FXPOI, it is also intended to promote the coordination and collaboration of research among other federal agencies, advocacy groups, and private partners. It is the intent of the working groups and the FXRCG to share the Research Plan with interested agencies and organizations.

The *Research Plan on Fragile X Syndrome and Associated Disorders* will also serve as a means of communicating scientific priorities to the research community. The Plan will be publicized broadly and made available on the NICHD Web site. One of the great strengths in the FXS and associated disorders research fields is the wealth of researchers proposing and performing innovative research. It is intended that this document will further stimulate new investigator-initiated applications and attract new investigators to the field.

As the NIH and other federal agencies, advocacy, and private partners work together to achieve the goals and objective in this Research Plan, the FXRCG will continue to function in a coordinating capacity to identify and facilitate future collaborative research efforts.

APPENDIX A: NIH-SUPPORTED *FMR1* GENE/FRAGILE X RESEARCH: A SELECTED BIBLIOGRAPHY

The following citations resulted from a search of MEDLINE, the premier biomedical literature database of the National Library of Medicine. The following terms were used: Fragile X syndrome; FXS; Fragile X Tremor/Ataxia; FXTAS; Fragile X Associated Ovarian Insufficiency; FXPOI; FXPOF; Fragile X Mental Retardation 1 gene; *FMR1*; *FMR1* protein; Research Support, NIH; Extramural.

The keyword [Research Support, NIH] and publication type [Extramural] is the designation for extramural research funded by the National Institutes of Health. This keyword was introduced in 2005.

Publications derived from NIH funded research in scientific journals indexed by PubMed.

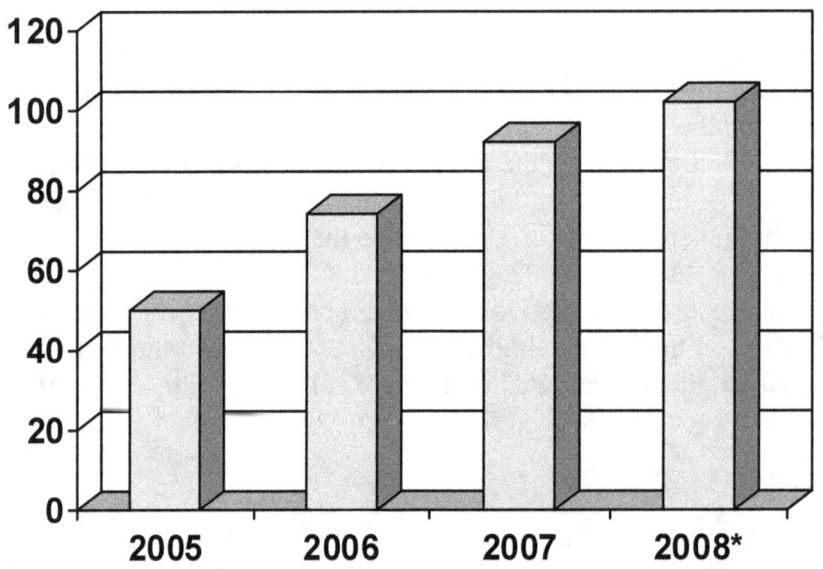

*estimated, based on six months

2008

Aguilar, D., et al., *A quantitative assessment of tremor and ataxia in FMR1 premutation carriers using CATSYS.* Am J Med Genet A, 2008. **146A**(5): p. 629-35.

Allen, E.G., et al., *Detection of early FXTAS motor symptoms using the CATSYS computerised neuromotor test battery.* J Med Genet, 2008. **45**(5): p. 290-7.

Amiri, K., R.J. Hagerman, and P.J. Hagerman, *Fragile X-associated tremor/ataxia syndrome: an aging face of the fragile X gene.* Arch Neurol, 2008. **65**(1): p. 19-25.

Amos Wilson, J., et al., *Consensus characterization of 16 FMR1 reference materials: a consortium study.* J Mol Diagn, 2008. **10**(1): p. 2-12.

Angkustsiri, K., et al., *Fragile X syndrome with anxiety disorder and exceptional verbal intelligence.* Am J Med Genet A, 2008. **146**(3): p. 376-9.

Bailey, D.B., Jr., et al., *Child and genetic variables associated with maternal adaptation to fragile X syndrome: a multidimensional analysis.* Am J Med Genet A, 2008. **146A**(6): p. 720-9.

Bailey, D.B., Jr., et al., *Ethical, legal, and social concerns about expanded newborn screening: fragile X syndrome as a prototype for emerging issues.* Pediatrics, 2008. **121**(3): p. e693-704.

Baranek, G.T., et al., *Developmental trajectories and correlates of sensory processing in young boys with fragile X syndrome.* Phys Occup Ther Pediatr, 2008. **28**(1): p. 79-98.

Bear, M.F., et al., *Fragile X: translation in action.* Neuropsychopharmacology, 2008. **33**(1): p. 84-7.

Bhattacharyya, A., et al., *Normal Neurogenesis but Abnormal Gene Expression in Human Fragile X Cortical Progenitor Cells.* Stem Cells Dev, 2008. **17**(1): p. 107-17.

Brodkin, E.S., *Social behavior phenotypes in fragile X syndrome, autism, and the Fmr1 knockout mouse: theoretical comment on McNaughton et al. (2008).* Behav Neurosci, 2008. **122**(2): p. 483-9.

Chang, S., et al., *Identification of small molecules rescuing fragile X syndrome phenotypes in Drosophila.* Nat Chem Biol, 2008. **4**(4): p. 256-63.

Coffee, B., et al., *Mosaic FMR1 deletion causes fragile X syndrome and can lead to molecular misdiagnosis: a case report and review of the literature.* Am J Med Genet A, 2008. **146A**(10): p. 1358-67.

Coffey, S.M., et al., *Expanded clinical phenotype of women with the FMR1 premutation.* Am J Med Genet A, 2008. **146A**(8): p. 1009-16.

Cornish, K.M., et al., *Age-dependent cognitive changes in carriers of the fragile X syndrome.* Cortex, 2008. **44**(6): p. 628-36.

de Vrij, F.M., et al., *Rescue of behavioral phenotype and neuronal protrusion morphology in Fmr1 KO mice.* Neurobiol Dis, 2008. **31**(1): p. 127-32.

Dictenberg, J.B., et al., *A direct role for FMRP in activity-dependent dendritic mRNA transport links filopodial-spine morphogenesis to fragile X syndrome.* Dev Cell, 2008. **14**(6): p. 926-39.

Dolen, G. and M.F. Bear, *Role for metabotropic glutamate receptor 5 (mGluR5) in the pathogenesis of fragile X syndrome.* J Physiol, 2008. **586**(6): p. 1503-8.

Gao, F.B., *Posttranscriptional control of neuronal development by microRNA networks.* Trends Neurosci, 2008. **31**(1): p. 20-6.

Garcia-Nonell, C., et al., *Secondary medical diagnosis in fragile X syndrome with and without autism spectrum disorder.* Am J Med Genet A, 2008. **146A**(15): p. 1911-6.

Gothelf, D., et al., *Neuroanatomy of fragile X syndrome is associated with aberrant behavior and the fragile X mental retardation protein (FMRP).* Ann Neurol, 2008. **63**(1): p. 40-51.

Grigsby, J., et al., *Cognitive profile of fragile X premutation carriers with and without fragile X-associated tremor/ataxia syndrome.* Neuropsychology, 2008. **22**(1): p. 48-60.

Hessl, D., et al., *Brief report: aggression and stereotypic behavior in males with fragile X syndrome--moderating secondary genes in a "single gene" disorder.* J Autism Dev Disord, 2008. **38**(1): p. 184-9.

Hooper, S.R., et al., *Executive functions in young males with fragile X syndrome in comparison to mental age-matched controls: baseline findings from a longitudinal study.* Neuropsychology, 2008. **22**(1): p. 36-47.

Iacoangeli, A., et al., *On BC1 RNA and the fragile X mental retardation protein.* Proc Natl Acad Sci U S A, 2008. **105**(2): p. 734-9.

Jenkins, E.C., et al., *Reduced telomere length in older men with premutation alleles of the fragile X mental retardation 1 gene.* Am J Med Genet A, 2008. **146A**(12): p. 1543-6.

Jiang, Y.H., et al., *Genomic analysis of the chromosome 15q11-q13 Prader-Willi syndrome region and characterization of transcripts for GOLGA8E and WHCD1L1 from the proximal breakpoint region.* BMC Genomics, 2008. **9**: p. 50.

Kim, S.H., et al., *Aberrant early-phase ERK inactivation impedes neuronal function in fragile X syndrome.* Proc Natl Acad Sci U S A, 2008. **105**(11): p. 4429-34.

Leehey, M.A., et al., *FMR1 CGG repeat length predicts motor dysfunction in premutation carriers.* Neurology, 2008. **70**(16 Pt 2): p. 1397-402.

Loesch, D.Z., et al., *A low symptomatic form of neurodegeneration in younger carriers of the FMR1 premutation, manifesting typical radiological changes.* J Med Genet, 2008. **45**(3): p. 179-81.

McConkie-Rosell, A., et al., *Living with genetic risk: effect on adolescent self-concept.* Am J Med Genet C Semin Med Genet, 2008. **148C**(1): p. 56-69.

McNaughton, C.H., et al., *Evidence for social anxiety and impaired social cognition in a mouse model of fragile X syndrome.* Behav Neurosci, 2008. **122**(2): p. 293-300.

Mili, S., K. Moissoglu, and I.G. Macara, *Genome-wide screen reveals APC-associated RNAs enriched in cell protrusions.* Nature, 2008. **453**(7191): p. 115-9.

Moon, J., et al., *A mouse model of fragile X syndrome exhibits heightened arousal and/or emotion following errors or reversal of contingencies.* Dev Psychobiol, 2008. **50**(5): p. 473-85.

Moy, S.S. and J.J. Nadler, *Advances in behavioral genetics: mouse models of autism.* Mol Psychiatry, 2008. **13**(1): p. 4-26.

Murphy, M.M. and M.M. Mazzocco, *Rote numeric skills may mask underlying mathematical disabilities in girls with fragile x syndrome.* Dev Neuropsychol, 2008. **33**(3): p. 345-64.

Murphy, M.M. and M.M. Mazzocco, *Mathematics learning disabilities in girls with fragile X or Turner syndrome during late elementary school.* J Learn Disabil, 2008. **41**(1): p. 29-46.

Nakayama, S., et al., *Role of the WWOX gene, encompassing fragile region FRA16D, in suppression of pancreatic carcinoma cells.* Cancer Sci, 2008. **99**(7): p. 1370-6.

Park, S., et al., *Elongation factor 2 and fragile X mental retardation protein control the dynamic translation of Arc/Arg3.1 essential for mGluR-LTD.* Neuron, 2008. **59**(1): p. 70-83.

Price, J.R., et al., *Syntactic complexity during conversation of boys with fragile X syndrome and Down syndrome.* J Speech Lang Hear Res, 2008. **51**(1): p. 3-15.

Roberts, J., et al., *Arousal modulation in females with fragile X or Turner syndrome.* J Autism Dev Disord, 2008. **38**(1): p. 20-7.

Rohr, J., et al., *Anti-Mullerian hormone indicates early ovarian decline in fragile X mental retardation (FMR1) premutation carriers: a preliminary study.* Hum Reprod, 2008. **23**(5): p. 1220-5.

Ronesi, J.A. and K.M. Huber, *Homer interactions are necessary for metabotropic glutamate receptor-induced long-term depression and translational activation.* J Neurosci, 2008. **28**(2): p. 543-7.

Shan, G., S. Xu, and P. Jin, *FXTAS: a bad RNA and a hope for a cure.* Expert Opin Biol Ther, 2008. **8**(3): p. 249-53.

Soontarapornchai, K., et al., *Abnormal nerve conduction features in fragile X premutation carriers.* Arch Neurol, 2008. **65**(4): p. 495-8.

Sulkowski, G.M. and L.M. Kaufman, *Oculomotor abnormalities in a patient with fragile X-associated tremor/ataxia syndrome.* J AAPOS, 2008. **12**(2): p. 195-6.

Tassone, F., et al., *A rapid polymerase chain reaction-based screening method for identification of all expanded alleles of the fragile X (FMR1) gene in newborn and high-risk populations.* J Mol Diagn, 2008. **10**(1): p. 43-9.

Tessier, C.R. and K. Broadie, *Drosophila fragile X mental retardation protein developmentally regulates activity-dependent axon pruning.* Development, 2008. **135**(8): p. 1547-57.

Wirojanan, J., et al., *A girl with fragile X premutation from sperm donation.* Am J Med Genet A, 2008. **146**(7): p. 888-92.

Wirojanan, J., et al., *Two boys with fragile x syndrome and hepatic tumors.* J Pediatr Hematol Oncol, 2008. **30**(3): p. 239-41.

Zhang, J., et al., *Fragile X-related proteins regulate mammalian circadian behavioral rhythms.* Am J Hum Genet, 2008. **83**(1): p. 43-52.

2007

Abbeduto, L., N. Brady, and S.T. Kover, *Language development and fragile X syndrome: profiles, syndrome-specificity, and within-syndrome differences.* Ment Retard Dev Disabil Res Rev, 2007. **13**(1): p. 36-46.

Adams, J.S., et al., *Volumetric brain changes in females with fragile X-associated tremor/ataxia syndrome (FXTAS).* Neurology, 2007. **69**(9): p. 851-9.

Allen, E.G., et al., *Examination of reproductive aging milestones among women who carry the FMR1 premutation.* Hum Reprod, 2007. **22**(8): p. 2142-52.

Anido, A., L.M. Carlson, and S.L. Sherman, *Attitudes toward fragile X mutation carrier testing from women identified in a general population survey.* J Genet Couns, 2007. **16**(1): p. 97-104.

Banerjee, P., et al., *Substitution of critical isoleucines in the KH domains of Drosophila fragile X protein results in partial loss-of-function phenotypes.* Genetics, 2007. **175**(3): p. 1241-50.

Berry-Kravis, E., et al., *Neuropathic features in fragile X premutation carriers.* Am J Med Genet A, 2007. **143**(1): p. 19-26.

Bourgeois, J.A., et al., *Cognitive, anxiety and mood disorders in the fragile X-associated tremor/ataxia syndrome.* Gen Hosp Psychiatry, 2007. **29**(4): p. 349-56.

Brouwer, J.R., et al., *Elevated Fmr1 mRNA levels and reduced protein expression in a mouse model with an unmethylated Fragile X full mutation.* Exp Cell Res, 2007. **313**(2): p. 244-53.

Brylawski, B.P., et al., *Mapping of an origin of DNA replication in the promoter of fragile X gene FMR1.* Exp Mol Pathol, 2007. **82**(2): p. 190-6.

Chang, T.C. and J.T. Mendell, *microRNAs in vertebrate physiology and human disease.* Annu Rev Genomics Hum Genet, 2007. **8**: p. 215-39.

Chiosea, S., et al., *Overexpression of Dicer in precursor lesions of lung adenocarcinoma.* Cancer Res, 2007. **67**(5): p. 2345-50.

Chiu, S., et al., *Early acceleration of head circumference in children with fragile x syndrome and autism.* J Dev Behav Pediatr, 2007. **28**(1): p. 31-5.

Clifford, S., et al., *Autism spectrum phenotype in males and females with fragile X full mutation and premutation.* J Autism Dev Disord, 2007. **37**(4): p. 738-47.

Cornish, K., G. Scerif, and A. Karmiloff-Smith, *Tracing syndrome-specific trajectories of attention across the lifespan.* Cortex, 2007. **43**(6): p. 672-85.

Dias, E.P., et al., *Association between decreased WWOX protein expression and thyroid cancer development.* Thyroid, 2007. **17**(11): p. 1055-9.

Dolen, G., et al., *Correction of fragile X syndrome in mice.* Neuron, 2007. **56**(6): p. 955-62.

Duan, P., et al., *Generation of polyclonal antiserum for the detection of methylarginine proteins.* J Immunol Methods, 2007. **320**(1-2): p. 132-42.

Durkin, S.G. and T.W. Glover, *Chromosome fragile sites.* Annu Rev Genet, 2007. **41**: p. 169-92.

Dykens, E.M. and R.M. Hodapp, *Three steps toward improving the measurement of behavior in behavioral phenotype research.* Child Adolesc Psychiatr Clin N Am, 2007. **16**(3): p. 617-30.

Fidler, D.J., A. Philofsky, and S.L. Hepburn, *Language phenotypes and intervention planning: bridging research and practice.* Ment Retard Dev Disabil Res Rev, 2007. **13**(1): p. 47-57.

Freudenreich, C.H., *Chromosome fragility: molecular mechanisms and cellular consequences.* Front Biosci, 2007. **12**: p. 4911-24.

Giorgi, C., et al., *The EJC factor eIF4AIII modulates synaptic strength and neuronal protein expression.* Cell, 2007. **130**(1): p. 179-91.

Govaerts, L.C., et al., *Exceptional good cognitive and phenotypic profile in a male carrying a mosaic mutation in the FMR1 gene.* Clin Genet, 2007. **72**(2): p. 138-44.

Gray, S.J., et al., *An origin of DNA replication in the promoter region of the human fragile X mental retardation (FMR1) gene.* Mol Cell Biol, 2007. **27**(2): p. 426-37.

Greco, C.M., et al., *Testicular and pituitary inclusion formation in fragile X associated tremor/ataxia syndrome.* J Urol, 2007. **177**(4): p. 1434-7.

Grigsby, J., et al., *Impairment of executive cognitive functioning in males with fragile X-associated tremor/ataxia syndrome.* Mov Disord, 2007. **22**(5): p. 645-50.

Hagerman, P.J. and R.J. Hagerman, *Fragile X-associated tremor/ataxia syndrome--an older face of the fragile X gene.* Nat Clin Pract Neurol, 2007. **3**(2): p. 107-12.

Hagerman, R.J., et al., *Neuropathy as a presenting feature in fragile X-associated tremor/ataxia syndrome.* Am J Med Genet A, 2007. **143A**(19): p. 2256-60.

Hall, S.S., D.D. Burns, and A.L. Reiss, *Modeling family dynamics in children with fragile x syndrome.* J Abnorm Child Psychol, 2007. **35**(1): p. 29-42.

Hanson, J.E. and D.V. Madison, *Presynaptic FMR1 genotype influences the degree of synaptic connectivity in a mosaic mouse model of fragile X syndrome.* J Neurosci, 2007. **27**(15): p. 4014-8.

Hayashi, M.L., et al., *Inhibition of p21-activated kinase rescues symptoms of fragile X syndrome in mice.* Proc Natl Acad Sci U S A, 2007. **104**(27): p. 11489-94.

Head, L.S. and L. Abbeduto, *Recognizing the role of parents in developmental outcomes: a systems approach to evaluating the child with developmental disabilities.* Ment Retard Dev Disabil Res Rev, 2007. **13**(4): p. 293-301.

Hessl, D., et al., *Amygdala dysfunction in men with the fragile X premutation.* Brain, 2007. **130**(Pt 2): p. 404-16.

Hoeft, F., et al., *Fronto-striatal dysfunction and potential compensatory mechanisms in male adolescents with fragile X syndrome.* Hum Brain Mapp, 2007. **28**(6): p. 543-54.

Jacquemont, S., et al., *Fragile-X syndrome and fragile X-associated tremor/ataxia syndrome: two faces of FMR1.* Lancet Neurol, 2007. **6**(1): p. 45-55.

Jin, P., et al., *Pur alpha binds to rCGG repeats and modulates repeat-mediated neurodegeneration in a Drosophila model of fragile X tremor/ataxia syndrome.* Neuron, 2007. **55**(4): p. 556-64.

Jung, J. and N. Bonini, *CREB-binding protein modulates repeat instability in a Drosophila model for polyQ disease.* Science, 2007. **315**(5820): p. 1857-9.

Keller-Bell, Y.D. and L. Abbeduto, *Narrative development in adolescents and young adults with fragile x syndrome.* Am J Ment Retard, 2007. **112**(4): p. 289-99.

Kelley, D.J., et al., *The cyclic AMP cascade is altered in the fragile X nervous system.* PLoS ONE, 2007. **2**(9): p. e931.

Kosmider, B. and R.D. Wells, *Fragile X repeats are potent inducers of complex, multiple site rearrangements in flanking sequences in Escherichia coli.* DNA Repair (Amst), 2007.

6(12): p. 1850-63.

Ladd, P.D., et al., *An antisense transcript spanning the CGG repeat region of FMR1 is upregulated in premutation carriers but silenced in full mutation individuals.* Hum Mol Genet, 2007. **16**(24): p. 3174-87.

Lasker, A.G., M.M. Mazzocco, and D.S. Zee, *Ocular motor indicators of executive dysfunction in fragile X and Turner syndromes.* Brain Cogn, 2007. **63**(3): p. 203-20.

Lauterborn, J.C., et al., *Brain-derived neurotrophic factor rescues synaptic plasticity in a mouse model of fragile X syndrome.* J Neurosci, 2007. **27**(40): p. 10685-94.

Lee, A.D., et al., *3D pattern of brain abnormalities in Fragile X syndrome visualized using tensor-based morphometry.* Neuroimage, 2007. **34**(3): p. 924-38.

Lee, H., et al., *Regulation of the sodium/sulfate co-transporter by farnesoid X receptor alpha.* J Biol Chem, 2007. **282**(30): p. 21653-61.

Leehey, M.A., et al., *Progression of tremor and ataxia in male carriers of the FMR1 premutation.* Mov Disord, 2007. **22**(2): p. 203-6.

Loesch, D.Z., et al., *Molecular and cognitive predictors of the continuum of autistic behaviours in fragile X.* Neurosci Biobehav Rev, 2007. **31**(3): p. 315-26.

Loesch, D.Z., et al., *Transcript levels of the intermediate size or grey zone fragile X mental retardation 1 alleles are raised, and correlate with the number of CGG repeats.* J Med Genet, 2007. **44**(3): p. 200-4.

Loesch, D.Z., et al., *Tremor/ataxia syndrome and fragile X premutation: diagnostic caveats.* J Clin Neurosci, 2007. **14**(3): p. 245-8.

McCloskey, M.L., et al., *Encoding PCR products with batch-stamps and barcodes.* Biochem Genet, 2007. **45**(11-12): p. 761-7.

Menon, L. and M.R. Mihailescu, *Interactions of the G quartet forming semaphorin 3F RNA with the RGG box domain of the fragile X protein family.* Nucleic Acids Res, 2007. **35**(16): p. 5379-92.

Moser, J.J., et al., *Markers of mRNA stabilization and degradation, and RNAi within astrocytoma GW bodies.* J Neurosci Res, 2007. **85**(16): p. 3619-31.

Muddashetty, R.S., et al., *Dysregulated metabotropic glutamate receptor-dependent translation of AMPA receptor and postsynaptic density-95 mRNAs at synapses in a mouse model of fragile X syndrome.* J Neurosci, 2007. **27**(20): p. 5338-48.

Muller, R.A., *The study of autism as a distributed disorder.* Ment Retard Dev Disabil Res Rev, 2007. **13**(1): p. 85-95.

Murphy, M.M. and L. Abbeduto, *Gender differences in repetitive language in fragile X syndrome.* J Intellect Disabil Res, 2007. **51**(Pt 5): p. 387-400.

Murphy, M.M., et al., *Contribution of social and information-processing factors to eye-gaze avoidance in fragile X syndrome.* Am J Ment Retard, 2007. **112**(5): p. 349-60.

Nakamoto, M., et al., *Fragile X mental retardation protein deficiency leads to excessive mGluR5-dependent internalization of AMPA receptors.* Proc Natl Acad Sci U S A, 2007.

104(39): p. 15537-42.

Narayanan, U., et al., *FMRP phosphorylation reveals an immediate-early signaling pathway triggered by group I mGluR and mediated by PP2A.* J Neurosci, 2007. **27**(52): p. 14349-57.

Nishimura, Y., et al., *Genome-wide expression profiling of lymphoblastoid cell lines distinguishes different forms of autism and reveals shared pathways.* Hum Mol Genet, 2007. **16**(14): p. 1682-98.

Nowicki, S.T., et al., *The Prader-Willi phenotype of fragile X syndrome.* J Dev Behav Pediatr, 2007. **28**(2): p. 133-8.

Okou, D.T., et al., *Microarray-based genomic selection for high-throughput resequencing.* Nat Methods, 2007. **4**(11): p. 907-9.

Orr, H.T. and H.Y. Zoghbi, *Trinucleotide repeat disorders.* Annu Rev Neurosci, 2007. **30**: p. 575-621.

Pan, L. and K.S. Broadie, *Drosophila fragile X mental retardation protein and metabotropic glutamate receptor A convergently regulate the synaptic ratio of ionotropic glutamate receptor subclasses.* J Neurosci, 2007. **27**(45): p. 12378-89.

Pfeiffer, B.E. and K.M. Huber, *Fragile X mental retardation protein induces synapse loss through acute postsynaptic translational regulation.* J Neurosci, 2007. **27**(12): p. 3120-30.

Price, T.J., et al., *Decreased nociceptive sensitization in mice lacking the fragile X mental retardation protein: role of mGluR1/5 and mTOR.* J Neurosci, 2007. **27**(51): p. 13958-67.

Probst, F.J., et al., *Chromosomal microarray analysis (CMA) detects a large X chromosome deletion including FMR1, FMR2, and IDS in a female patient with mental retardation.* Am J Med Genet A, 2007. **143A**(12): p. 1358-65.

Reiss, A.L. and S.S. Hall, *Fragile X syndrome: assessment and treatment implications.* Child Adolesc Psychiatr Clin N Am, 2007. **16**(3): p. 663-75.

Roberts, J., et al., *Discourse skills of boys with fragile X syndrome in comparison to boys with Down syndrome.* J Speech Lang Hear Res, 2007. **50**(2): p. 475-92.

Roberts, J., et al., *Receptive vocabulary, expressive vocabulary, and speech production of boys with fragile X syndrome in comparison to boys with down syndrome.* Am J Ment Retard, 2007. **112**(3): p. 177-93.

Roberts, J.E., et al., *Expressive language during conversational speech in boys with fragile X syndrome.* Am J Ment Retard, 2007. **112**(1): p. 1-17.

Roberts, J.E., et al., *Social approach and autistic behavior in children with fragile X syndrome.* J Autism Dev Disord, 2007. **37**(9): p. 1748-60.

Scambler, D.J., et al., *A preliminary study of screening for risk of autism in children with fragile X syndrome: testing two risk cut-offs for the Checklist for Autism in Toddlers.* J Intellect Disabil Res, 2007. **51**(Pt 4): p. 269-76.

Scerif, G., et al., *Delineation of early attentional control difficulties in fragile X syndrome: focus on neurocomputational changes.* Neuropsychologia, 2007. **45**(8): p. 1889-98.

Selby, L., C. Zhang, and Q.Q. Sun, *Major defects in neocortical GABAergic inhibitory circuits in mice lacking the fragile X mental retardation protein.* Neurosci Lett, 2007. **412**(3): p. 227-32.

Sofola, O.A., et al., *Argonaute-2-dependent rescue of a Drosophila model of FXTAS by FRAXE premutation repeat.* Hum Mol Genet, 2007. **16**(19): p. 2326-32.

Sofola, O.A., et al., *RNA-binding proteins hnRNP A2/B1 and CUGBP1 suppress fragile X CGG premutation repeat-induced neurodegeneration in a Drosophila model of FXTAS.* Neuron, 2007. **55**(4): p. 565-71.

Solomon, M., et al., *A genetic etiology of pervasive developmental disorder guides treatment.* Am J Psychiatry, 2007. **164**(4): p. 575-80.

Sullivan, K., et al., *Sustained attention and response inhibition in boys with fragile X syndrome: measures of continuous performance.* Am J Med Genet B Neuropsychiatr Genet, 2007. **144B**(4): p. 517-32.

Sullivan, K., S. Hooper, and D. Hatton, *Behavioural equivalents of anxiety in children with fragile X syndrome: parent and teacher report.* J Intellect Disabil Res, 2007. **51**(Pt 1): p. 54-65.

Taffe, J.R., et al., *Short form of the developmental behaviour checklist.* Am J Ment Retard, 2007. **112**(1): p. 31-9.

Tassone, F., et al., *CGG repeat length correlates with age of onset of motor signs of the fragile X-associated tremor/ataxia syndrome (FXTAS).* Am J Med Genet B Neuropsychiatr Genet, 2007. **144B**(4): p. 566-9.

Tassone, F., et al., *Elevated FMR1 mRNA in premutation carriers is due to increased transcription.* RNA, 2007. **13**(4): p. 555-62.

Vasudevan, S. and J.A. Steitz, *AU-rich-element-mediated upregulation of translation by FXR1 and Argonaute 2.* Cell, 2007. **128**(6): p. 1105-18.

Vasudevan, S., Y. Tong, and J.A. Steitz, *Switching from repression to activation: microRNAs can up-regulate translation.* Science, 2007. **318**(5858): p. 1931-4.

Volk, L.J., et al., *Multiple Gq-coupled receptors converge on a common protein synthesis-dependent long-term depression that is affected in fragile X syndrome mental retardation.* J Neurosci, 2007. **27**(43): p. 11624-34.

Wang, W., et al., *RNA transport and localized protein synthesis in neurological disorders and neural repair.* Dev Neurobiol, 2007. **67**(9): p. 1166-82.

Westmark, C.J. and J.S. Malter, *FMRP mediates mGluR5-dependent translation of amyloid precursor protein.* PLoS Biol, 2007. **5**(3): p. e52.

Wilson, B.M. and C.L. Cox, *Absence of metabotropic glutamate receptor-mediated plasticity in the neocortex of fragile X mice.* Proc Natl Acad Sci U S A, 2007. **104**(7): p. 2454-9.

Yan, Y. and K. Broadie, *In vivo assay of presynaptic microtubule cytoskeleton dynamics in Drosophila.* J Neurosci Methods, 2007. **162**(1-2): p. 198-205.

Yang, L., et al., *Fragile X mental retardation protein modulates the fate of germline stem cells in Drosophila.* Hum Mol Genet, 2007. **16**(15): p. 1814-20.

Zhang, H. and C.H. Freudenreich, *An AT-rich sequence in human common fragile site FRA16D causes fork stalling and chromosome breakage in S. cerevisiae.* Mol Cell, 2007. **27**(3): p. 367-79.

Zhu, M. and R.S. Weiss, *Increased common fragile site expression, cell proliferation defects, and apoptosis following conditional inactivation of mouse Hus1 in primary cultured cells.* Mol Biol Cell, 2007. **18**(3): p. 1044-55.

Zumwalt, M., et al., *Secondary structure and dynamics of the r(CGG) repeat in the mRNA of the fragile X mental retardation 1 (FMR1) gene.* RNA Biol, 2007. **4**(2): p. 93-100.

2006

Abbeduto, L., et al., *Collaboration in referential communication: comparison of youth with down syndrome or fragile X syndrome.* Am J Ment Retard, 2006. **111**(3): p. 170-83.

Admire, A., et al., *Cycles of chromosome instability are associated with a fragile site and are increased by defects in DNA replication and checkpoint controls in yeast.* Genes Dev, 2006. **20**(2): p. 159-73.

Albertson, D.G., *Gene amplification in cancer.* Trends Genet, 2006. **22**(8): p. 447-55.

Antar, L.N., et al., *Local functions for FMRP in axon growth cone motility and activity-dependent regulation of filopodia and spine synapses.* Mol Cell Neurosci, 2006. **32**(1-2): p. 37-48.

Bacalman, S., et al., *Psychiatric phenotype of the fragile X-associated tremor/ataxia syndrome (FXTAS) in males: newly described fronto-subcortical dementia.* J Clin Psychiatry, 2006. **67**(1): p. 87-94.

Barbee, S.A., et al., *Staufen- and FMRP-containing neuronal RNPs are structurally and functionally related to somatic P bodies.* Neuron, 2006. **52**(6): p. 997-1009.

Barnes, E.F., et al., *A comparison of oral structure and oral-motor function in young males with fragile X syndrome and Down syndrome.* J Speech Lang Hear Res, 2006. **49**(4): p. 903-17.

Bourgeois, J.A., et al., *Dementia with mood symptoms in a fragile X premutation carrier with the fragile X-associated tremor/ataxia syndrome: clinical intervention with donepezil and venlafaxine.* J Neuropsychiatry Clin Neurosci, 2006. **18**(2): p. 171-7.

Brady, N., et al., *Communication in young children with fragile X syndrome: a qualitative study of mothers' perspectives.* Am J Speech Lang Pathol, 2006. **15**(4): p. 353-64.

Brennan, F.X., D.S. Albeck, and R. Paylor, *Fmr1 knockout mice are impaired in a leverpress escape/avoidance task.* Genes Brain Behav, 2006. **5**(6): p. 467-71.

Budimirovic, D.B., et al., *Autism spectrum disorder in Fragile X syndrome: differential contribution of adaptive socialization and social withdrawal.* Am J Med Genet A, 2006. **140A**(17): p. 1814-26.

Chmiel, N.H., D.C. Rio, and J.A. Doudna, *Distinct contributions of KH domains to substrate binding affinity of Drosophila P-element somatic inhibitor protein.* RNA, 2006. **12**(2): p.

283-91.

Cohen, S., et al., *Molecular and imaging correlates of the fragile X-associated tremor/ataxia syndrome.* Neurology, 2006. **67**(8): p. 1426-31.

Deshpande, G., G. Calhoun, and P. Schedl, *The drosophila fragile X protein dFMR1 is required during early embryogenesis for pole cell formation and rapid nuclear division cycles.* Genetics, 2006. **174**(3): p. 1287-98.

Dickson, C.A., et al., *Matching-to-sample assessment of stimulus overselectivity in students with intellectual disabilities.* Am J Ment Retard, 2006. **111**(6): p. 447-53.

Dolzhanskaya, N., et al., *Methylation regulates the intracellular protein-protein and protein-RNA interactions of FMRP.* J Cell Sci, 2006. **119**(Pt 9): p. 1933-46.

Durkin, S.G., et al., *Depletion of CHK1, but not CHK2, induces chromosomal instability and breaks at common fragile sites.* Oncogene, 2006. **25**(32): p. 4381-8.

Farzin, F., et al., *Autism spectrum disorders and attention-deficit/hyperactivity disorder in boys with the fragile X premutation.* J Dev Behav Pediatr, 2006. **27**(2 Suppl): p. S137-44.

Garber, K., et al., *Transcription, translation and fragile X syndrome.* Curr Opin Genet Dev, 2006. **16**(3): p. 270-5.

Gheldof, N., T.M. Tabuchi, and J. Dekker, *The active FMR1 promoter is associated with a large domain of altered chromatin conformation with embedded local histone modifications.* Proc Natl Acad Sci U S A, 2006. **103**(33): p. 12463-8.

Glover, T.W., *Common fragile sites.* Cancer Lett, 2006. **232**(1): p. 4-12.

Greco, C.M., et al., *Neuropathology of fragile X-associated tremor/ataxia syndrome (FXTAS).* Brain, 2006. **129**(Pt 1): p. 243-55.

Grigsby, J., et al., *Impairment in the cognitive functioning of men with fragile X-associated tremor/ataxia syndrome (FXTAS).* J Neurol Sci, 2006. **248**(1-2): p. 227-33.

Grigsby, J., et al., *Cognitive impairment in a 65-year-old male with the fragile X-associated tremor-ataxia syndrome (FXTAS).* Cogn Behav Neurol, 2006. **19**(3): p. 165-71.

Grossman, A.W., et al., *Local protein synthesis and spine morphogenesis: Fragile X syndrome and beyond.* J Neurosci, 2006. **26**(27): p. 7151-5.

Grossman, A.W., et al., *Hippocampal pyramidal cells in adult Fmr1 knockout mice exhibit an immature-appearing profile of dendritic spines.* Brain Res, 2006. **1084**(1): p. 158-64.

Hagerman, R.J., *Lessons from fragile X regarding neurobiology, autism, and neurodegeneration.* J Dev Behav Pediatr, 2006. **27**(1): p. 63-74.

Hall, D.A., et al., *Symptomatic treatment in the fragile X-associated tremor/ataxia syndrome.* Mov Disord, 2006. **21**(10): p. 1741-4.

Hall, D.A., et al., *Prevalence of FMR1 repeat expansions in movement disorders. A systematic review.* Neuroepidemiology, 2006. **26**(3): p. 151-5.

Hall, S., M. DeBernardis, and A. Reiss, *Social escape behaviors in children with fragile X syndrome.* J Autism Dev Disord, 2006. **36**(7): p. 935-47.

Hall, S.S., G.M. Debernardis, and A.L. Reiss, *The acquisition of stimulus equivalence in individuals with fragile X syndrome.* J Intellect Disabil Res, 2006. **50**(Pt 9): p. 643-51.

Hatton, D.D., et al., *Autistic behavior in children with fragile X syndrome: prevalence, stability, and the impact of FMRP.* Am J Med Genet A, 2006. **140A**(17): p. 1804-13.

Hessl, D., et al., *Social behavior and cortisol reactivity in children with fragile X syndrome.* J Child Psychol Psychiatry, 2006. **47**(6): p. 602-10.

Hiraki, S., et al., *Attitudes of genetic counselors towards expanding newborn screening and offering predictive genetic testing to children.* Am J Med Genet A, 2006. **140**(21): p. 2312-9.

Hou, L., et al., *Dynamic translational and proteasomal regulation of fragile X mental retardation protein controls mGluR-dependent long-term depression.* Neuron, 2006. **51**(4): p. 441-54.

Iliopoulos, D., et al., *Roles of FHIT and WWOX fragile genes in cancer.* Cancer Lett, 2006. **232**(1): p. 27-36.

Iwahashi, C.K., et al., *Protein composition of the intranuclear inclusions of FXTAS.* Brain, 2006. **129**(Pt 1): p. 256-71.

Jacquemont, S., et al., *Size bias of fragile X premutation alleles in late-onset movement disorders.* J Med Genet, 2006. **43**(10): p. 804-9.

Johnson, E.M., et al., *Role of Pur alpha in targeting mRNA to sites of translation in hippocampal neuronal dendrites.* J Neurosci Res, 2006. **83**(6): p. 929-43.

Kim, S.H., et al., *Fragile X mental retardation protein shifts between polyribosomes and stress granules after neuronal injury by arsenite stress or in vivo hippocampal electrode insertion.* J Neurosci, 2006. **26**(9): p. 2413-8.

Kosmider, B. and R.D. Wells, *Double-strand breaks in the myotonic dystrophy type 1 and the fragile X syndrome triplet repeat sequences induce different types of mutations in DNA flanking sequences in Escherichia coli.* Nucleic Acids Res, 2006. **34**(19): p. 5369-82.

Kuo, M.T., et al., *Association of fragile site-associated (FSA) gene expression with epithelial differentiation and tumor development.* Biochem Biophys Res Commun, 2006. **340**(3): p. 887-93.

Lewis, P., et al., *Cognitive, language and social-cognitive skills of individuals with fragile X syndrome with and without autism.* J Intellect Disabil Res, 2006. **50**(Pt 7): p. 532-45.

Lewis, P., et al., *Psychological well-being of mothers of youth with fragile X syndrome: syndrome specificity and within-syndrome variability.* J Intellect Disabil Res, 2006. **50**(Pt 12): p. 894-904.

Lightbody, A.A., S.S. Hall, and A.L. Reiss, *Chronological age, but not FMRP levels, predicts neuropsychological performance in girls with fragile X syndrome.* Am J Med Genet B Neuropsychiatr Genet, 2006. **141B**(5): p. 468-72.

Loat, C.S., et al., *Investigating the relationship between FMR1 allele length and cognitive ability in children: a subtle effect of the normal allele range on the normal ability range?* Ann Hum Genet, 2006. **70**(Pt 5): p. 555-65.

Louis, E., et al., *Parkinsonism, dysautonomia, and intranuclear inclusions in a fragile X carrier: a clinical-pathological study.* Mov Disord, 2006. **21**(3): p. 420-5.

Markham, J.A., et al., *Corticosterone response to acute stress in a mouse model of Fragile X syndrome.* Psychoneuroendocrinology, 2006. **31**(6): p. 781-5.

Mazzocco, M.M., N. Singh Bhatia, and K. Lesniak-Karpiak, *Visuospatial skills and their association with math performance in girls with fragile X or Turner syndrome.* Child Neuropsychol, 2006. **12**(2): p. 87-110.

Mazzocco, M.M., et al., *Language use in females with fragile X or Turner syndrome during brief initial social interactions.* J Dev Behav Pediatr, 2006. **27**(4): p. 319-28.

Megosh, H.B., et al., *The role of PIWI and the miRNA machinery in Drosophila germline determination.* Curr Biol, 2006. **16**(19): p. 1884-94.

Mientjes, E.J., et al., *The generation of a conditional Fmr1 knock out mouse model to study Fmrp function in vivo.* Neurobiol Dis, 2006. **21**(3): p. 549-55.

Miller, C.T., et al., *Genomic amplification of MET with boundaries within fragile site FRA7G and upregulation of MET pathways in esophageal adenocarcinoma.* Oncogene, 2006. **25**(3): p. 409-18.

Mirkin, S.M., *DNA structures, repeat expansions and human hereditary disorders.* Curr Opin Struct Biol, 2006. **16**(3): p. 351-8.

Monzo, K., et al., *Fragile X mental retardation protein controls trailer hitch expression and cleavage furrow formation in Drosophila embryos.* Proc Natl Acad Sci U S A, 2006. **103**(48): p. 18160-5.

Moon, J., et al., *Attentional dysfunction, impulsivity, and resistance to change in a mouse model of fragile X syndrome.* Behav Neurosci, 2006. **120**(6): p. 1367-79.

Murphy, M.M., et al., *Mathematics learning disability in girls with Turner syndrome or fragile X syndrome.* Brain Cogn, 2006. **61**(2): p. 195-210.

Nosyreva, E.D. and K.M. Huber, *Metabotropic receptor-dependent long-term depression persists in the absence of protein synthesis in the mouse model of fragile X syndrome.* J Neurophysiol, 2006. **95**(5): p. 3291-5.

Osborne, R.J. and C.A. Thornton, *RNA-dominant diseases.* Hum Mol Genet, 2006. **15 Spec No 2**: p. R162-9.

Parrini, E., et al., *Periventricular heterotopia: phenotypic heterogeneity and correlation with Filamin A mutations.* Brain, 2006. **129**(Pt 7): p. 1892-906.

Price, T.J., et al., *The RNA binding and transport proteins staufen and fragile X mental retardation protein are expressed by rat primary afferent neurons and localize to peripheral and central axons.* Neuroscience, 2006. **141**(4): p. 2107-16.

Ramos, D. and C.M. Aldaz, *WWOX, a chromosomal fragile site gene and its role in cancer.* Adv Exp Med Biol, 2006. **587**: p. 149-59.

Ranum, L.P. and T.A. Cooper, *RNA-mediated neuromuscular disorders.* Annu Rev Neurosci, 2006. **29**: p. 259-77.

Raveendranathan, M., et al, *Genome-wide replication profiles of S-phase checkpoint mutants reveal fragile sites in yeast.* EMBO J, 2006. **25**(15): p. 3627-39.

Smith, K.T., R.D. Nicholls, and D. Reines, *The gene encoding the fragile X RNA-binding protein is controlled by nuclear respiratory factor 2 and the CREB family of transcription factors.* Nucleic Acids Res, 2006. **34**(4): p. 1205-15.

Spencer, C.M., et al., *Exaggerated behavioral phenotypes in Fmr1/Fxr2 double knockout mice reveal a functional genetic interaction between Fragile X-related proteins.* Hum Mol Genet, 2006. **15**(12): p. 1984-94.

Stankiewicz, P., et al., *Minimal phenotype in a girl with trisomy 15q due to t(X;15)(q22.3;q11.2) translocation.* Am J Med Genet A, 2006. **140**(5): p. 442-52.

Stetler, A., et al., *Identification and characterization of the methyl arginines in the fragile X mental retardation protein Fmrp.* Hum Mol Genet, 2006. **15**(1): p. 87-96.

Sullivan, K., et al., *ADHD symptoms in children with FXS.* Am J Med Genet A, 2006. **140**(21): p. 2275-88.

Wang, Y.H., *Chromatin structure of human chromosomal fragile sites.* Cancer Lett, 2006. **232**(1): p. 70-8.

Wei, Y., et al., *Molecular cloning of Chinese hamster 1q31 chromosomal fragile site DNA that is important to mdr1 gene amplification reveals a novel gene whose expression is associated with spermatocyte and adipocyte differentiation.* Gene, 2006. **372**: p. 44-52.

Yun, S.W., et al., *Fmrp is required for the establishment of the startle response during the critical period of auditory development.* Brain Res, 2006. **1110**(1): p. 159-65.

Zajac, D.J., et al., *Articulation rate and vowel space characteristics of young males with fragile X syndrome: preliminary acoustic findings.* J Speech Lang Hear Res, 2006. **49**(5): p. 1147-55.

Zanotti, K.J., et al., *Thermodynamics of the fragile X mental retardation protein RGG box interactions with G quartet forming RNA.* Biochemistry, 2006. **45**(27): p. 8319-30.

2004-2005

Acharya, K., P.D. Ackerman, and L.F. Ross, *Pediatricians' attitudes toward expanding newborn screening.* Pediatrics, 2005. **116**(4): p. e476-84.

Allen, E.G., et al., *Examination of the effect of the polymorphic CGG repeat in the FMR1 gene on cognitive performance.* Behav Genet, 2005. **35**(4): p. 435-45.

Anido, A., et al., *Women's attitudes toward testing for fragile X carrier status: a qualitative analysis.* J Genet Couns, 2005. **14**(4): p. 295-306.

Antar, L.N., et al., *Localization of FMRP-associated mRNA granules and requirement of microtubules for activity-dependent trafficking in hippocampal neurons.* Genes Brain Behav, 2005. **4**(6): p. 350-9.

Arocena, D.G., et al., *Induction of inclusion formation and disruption of lamin A/C structure by premutation CGG-repeat RNA in human cultured neural cells.* Hum Mol Genet, 2005.

14(23): p. 3661-71.

Bear, M.F., *Therapeutic implications of the mGluR theory of fragile X mental retardation.* Genes Brain Behav, 2005. **4**(6): p. 393-8.

Bettencourt da Cruz, A., et al., *Disruption of the MAP1B-related protein FUTSCH leads to changes in the neuronal cytoskeleton, axonal transport defects, and progressive neurodegeneration in Drosophila.* Mol Biol Cell, 2005. **16**(5): p. 2433-42.

Biancalana, V., et al., *FMR1 premutations associated with fragile X-associated tremor/ataxia syndrome in multiple system atrophy.* Arch Neurol, 2005. **62**(6): p. 962-6.

Chuang, S.C., et al., *Prolonged epileptiform discharges induced by altered group I metabotropic glutamate receptor-mediated synaptic responses in hippocampal slices of a fragile X mouse model.* J Neurosci, 2005. **25**(35): p. 8048-55.

Coon, H., et al., *Evidence for linkage on chromosome 3q25-27 in a large autism extended pedigree.* Hum Hered, 2005. **60**(4): p. 220-6.

Corrigan, E.C., et al., *A woman with spontaneous premature ovarian failure gives birth to a child with fragile X syndrome.* Fertil Steril, 2005. **84**(5): p. 1508.

Darnell, J.C., et al., *Kissing complex RNAs mediate interaction between the Fragile-X mental retardation protein KH2 domain and brain polyribosomes.* Genes Dev, 2005. **19**(8): p. 903-18.

Darnell, J.C., O. Mostovetsky, and R.B. Darnell, *FMRP RNA targets: identification and validation.* Genes Brain Behav, 2005. **4**(6): p. 341-9.

Di Prospero, N.A. and K.H. Fischbeck, *Therapeutics development for triplet repeat expansion diseases.* Nat Rev Genet, 2005. **6**(10): p. 756-65.

Galvez, R. and W.T. Greenough, *Sequence of abnormal dendritic spine development in primary somatosensory cortex of a mouse model of the fragile X mental retardation syndrome.* Am J Med Genet A, 2005. **135**(2): p. 155-60.

Galvez, R., R.L. Smith, and W.T. Greenough, *Olfactory bulb mitral cell dendritic pruning abnormalities in a mouse model of the Fragile-X mental retardation syndrome: further support for FMRP's involvement in dendritic development.* Brain Res Dev Brain Res, 2005. **157**(2): p. 214-6.

Genereux, D.P., et al., *A population-epigenetic model to infer site-specific methylation rates from double-stranded DNA methylation patterns.* Proc Natl Acad Sci U S A, 2005. **102**(16): p. 5802-7.

Glover, T.W., et al., *Mechanisms of common fragile site instability.* Hum Mol Genet, 2005. **14 Spec No. 2**: p. R197-205.

Gothelf, D., et al., *The contribution of novel brain imaging techniques to understanding the neurobiology of mental retardation and developmental disabilities.* Ment Retard Dev Disabil Res Rev, 2005. **11**(4): p. 331-9.

Guler, G., et al., *Concordant loss of fragile gene expression early in breast cancer development.* Pathol Int, 2005. **55**(8): p. 471-8.

Hall, D.A., et al., *Initial diagnoses given to persons with the fragile X associated tremor/ataxia syndrome (FXTAS).* Neurology, 2005. **65**(2): p. 299-301.

Haydar, T.F., *Advanced microscopic imaging methods to investigate cortical development and the etiology of mental retardation.* Ment Retard Dev Disabil Res Rev, 2005. **11**(4): p. 303-16.

Hessl, D., et al., *Abnormal elevation of FMR1 mRNA is associated with psychological symptoms in individuals with the fragile X premutation.* Am J Med Genet B Neuropsychiatr Genet, 2005. **139B**(1): p. 115-21.

Howlett, N.G., et al., *The Fanconi anemia pathway is required for the DNA replication stress response and for the regulation of common fragile site stability.* Hum Mol Genet, 2005. **14**(5): p. 693-701.

Irwin, S.A., et al., *Fragile X mental retardation protein levels increase following complex environment exposure in rat brain regions undergoing active synaptogenesis.* Neurobiol Learn Mem, 2005. **83**(3): p. 180-7.

Jacquemont, S., et al., *Spastic paraparesis, cerebellar ataxia, and intention tremor: a severe variant of FXTAS?* J Med Genet, 2005. **42**(2): p. e14.

Kerber, K.A., et al., *Late-onset pure cerebellar ataxia: differentiating those with and without identifiable mutations.* J Neurol Sci, 2005. **238**(1-2): p. 41-5.

Kirk, J.W., M.M. Mazzocco, and S.T. Kover, *Assessing executive dysfunction in girls with fragile X or Turner syndrome using the Contingency Naming Test (CNT).* Dev Neuropsychol, 2005. **28**(3): p. 755-77.

Koekkoek, S.K., et al., *Deletion of FMR1 in Purkinje cells enhances parallel fiber LTD, enlarges spines, and attenuates cerebellar eyelid conditioning in Fragile X syndrome.* Neuron, 2005. **47**(3): p. 339-52.

Larson, J., et al., *Age-dependent and selective impairment of long-term potentiation in the anterior piriform cortex of mice lacking the fragile X mental retardation protein.* J Neurosci, 2005. **25**(41): p. 9460-9.

Lim, J.H., A.B. Booker, and J.R. Fallon, *Regulating fragile X gene transcription in the brain and beyond.* J Cell Physiol, 2005. **205**(2): p. 170-5.

Lim, J.H., et al., *AP-2alpha selectively regulates fragile X mental retardation-1 gene transcription during embryonic development.* Hum Mol Genet, 2005. **14**(14): p. 2027-34.

Lim, J.H., et al., *Developmental expression of Xenopus fragile X mental retardation-1 gene.* Int J Dev Biol, 2005. **49**(8): p. 981-4.

Loesch, D.Z., et al., *Evidence for, and a spectrum of, neurological involvement in carriers of the fragile X pre-mutation: FXTAS and beyond.* Clin Genet, 2005. **67**(5): p. 412-7.

Loesch, D.Z., et al., *Magnetic resonance imaging study in older fragile X premutation male carriers.* Ann Neurol, 2005. **58**(2): p. 326-30.

Lugli, G., et al., *Dicer and eIF2c are enriched at postsynaptic densities in adult mouse brain and are modified by neuronal activity in a calpain-dependent manner.* J Neurochem, 2005. **94**(4): p. 896-905.

McInnes, L.A., et al., *A genetic study of autism in Costa Rica: multiple variables affecting IQ scores observed in a preliminary sample of autistic cases.* BMC Psychiatry, 2005. **5**: p. 15.

McKinney, B.C., et al., *Dendritic spine abnormalities in the occipital cortex of C57BL/6 Fmr1 knockout mice.* Am J Med Genet B Neuropsychiatr Genet, 2005. **136B**(1): p. 98-102.

Mothersead, P.K., et al., *GRAND ROUNDS: an atypical progressive dementia in a male carrier of the fragile X premutation: an example of fragile X-associated tremor/ataxia syndrome.* Appl Neuropsychol, 2005. **12**(3): p. 169-78.

Musci, T.J. and A.B. Caughey, *Cost-effectiveness analysis of prenatal population-based fragile X carrier screening.* Am J Obstet Gynecol, 2005. **192**(6): p. 1905-12; discussion 1912-5.

Poehlmann, J., et al., *Family experiences associated with a child's diagnosis of fragile X or Down syndrome: evidence for disruption and resilience.* Ment Retard, 2005. **43**(4): p. 255-67.

Reeve, S.P., et al., *The Drosophila fragile X mental retardation protein controls actin dynamics by directly regulating profilin in the brain.* Curr Biol, 2005. **15**(12): p. 1156-63.

Restifo, L.L., *Mental retardation genes in drosophila: New approaches to understanding and treating developmental brain disorders.* Ment Retard Dev Disabil Res Rev, 2005. **11**(4): p. 286-94.

Restivo, L., et al., *Enriched environment promotes behavioral and morphological recovery in a mouse model for the fragile X syndrome.* Proc Natl Acad Sci U S A, 2005. **102**(32): p. 11557-62.

Roberts, J., et al., *Auditory brainstem responses in young males with Fragile X syndrome.* J Speech Lang Hear Res, 2005. **48**(2): p. 494-500.

Roberts, J., et al., *A comparison of phonological skills of boys with fragile X syndrome and Down syndrome.* J Speech Lang Hear Res, 2005. **48**(5): p. 980-95.

Roberts, J.E., et al., *Blink rate in boys with fragile X syndrome: preliminary evidence for altered dopamine function.* J Intellect Disabil Res, 2005. **49**(Pt 9): p. 647-56.

Rogers, S.J. and S. Ozonoff, *Annotation: what do we know about sensory dysfunction in autism? A critical review of the empirical evidence.* J Child Psychol Psychiatry, 2005. **46**(12): p. 1255-68.

Saluto, A., et al., *An enhanced polymerase chain reaction assay to detect pre- and full mutation alleles of the fragile X mental retardation 1 gene.* J Mol Diagn, 2005. **7**(5): p. 605-12.

Schwartz, M., et al., *Homologous recombination and nonhomologous end-joining repair pathways regulate fragile site stability.* Genes Dev, 2005. **19**(22): p. 2715-26.

Seixas, A.I., et al., *FXTAS, SCA10, and SCA17 in American patients with movement disorders.* Am J Med Genet A, 2005. **136**(1): p. 87-9.

Sullivan, A.K., et al., *Association of FMR1 repeat size with ovarian dysfunction.* Hum Reprod, 2005. **20**(2): p. 402-12.

Thavathiru, E., et al., *Expression of common chromosomal fragile site genes, WWOX/FRA16D and FHIT/FRA3B is downregulated by exposure to environmental carcinogens, UV, and BPDE but not by IR.* Mol Carcinog, 2005. **44**(3): p. 174-82.

Vanderklish, P.W. and G.M. Edelman, *Differential translation and fragile X syndrome.* Genes Brain Behav, 2005. **4**(6): p. 360-84.

Visootsak, J., et al., *Fragile X syndrome: an update and review for the primary pediatrician.* Clin Pediatr (Phila), 2005. **44**(5): p. 371-81.

Wang, H., et al., *Dendritic BC1 RNA in translational control mechanisms.* J Cell Biol, 2005. **171**(5): p. 811-21.

Willemsen, R., E. Mientjes, and B.A. Oostra, *FXTAS: a progressive neurologic syndrome associated with Fragile X premutation.* Curr Neurol Neurosci Rep, 2005. **5**(5): p. 405-10.

Yobb, T.M., et al., *Microduplication and triplication of 22q11.2: a highly variable syndrome.* Am J Hum Genet, 2005. **76**(5): p. 865-76.

Zhang, Y.Q., et al., *Protein expression profiling of the drosophila fragile X mutant brain reveals up-regulation of monoamine synthesis.* Mol Cell Proteomics, 2005. **4**(3): p. 278-90.

Gabel, L.A., et al., *Visual experience regulates transient expression and dendritic localization of fragile X mental retardation protein.* J Neurosci, 2004. **24**(47): p. 10579-83.

Tassone, F., C. Iwahashi, and P.J. Hagerman, *FMR1 RNA within the intranuclear inclusions of fragile X-associated tremor/ataxia syndrome (FXTAS).* RNA Biol, 2004. **1**(2): p. 103-5.